homeopathy

in essence

Andrew James

Series Editor: Nicola Jenkins

Hodder Arnold

A MEMBER OF THE HODDER HEADLINE GROUP

Orders: please contact Bookpoint Ltd, 130 Milton Park, Abingdon, Oxon OX14 4SB. Telephone: (44) 01235 827720.
Fax: (44) 01235 400454. Lines are open from 9.00 - 5.00, Monday to Saturday, with a 24-hour message answering service.
You can also order through our website www.hoddereducation.co.uk

If you have any comments to make about this, or any of our other titles, please send them to
educationenquiries@hodder.co.uk

British Library Cataloguing in Publication Data
A catalogue record for this title is available from the British Library

ISBN-10: 0 340 92692 9
ISBN-13: 978 0 340 92692 5

This Edition Published 2006
Impression number   10 9 8 7 6 5 4 3 2 1
Year   2010 2009 2008 2007 2006

Hodder Headline's policy is to use papers that are natural, renewable and recyclable products and made from wood
grown in sustainable forests. The logging and manufacturing processes are expected to conform to the environmental
regulations of the country of origin.

You should always consult a doctor for treatment of any ongoing serious medical condition or any undiagnosed condition.

Cover photo from Carl Drury
Printed in Great Britain by CPI Bath

acknowledgements

This book is dedicated with love to Mary, my mum.

With thanks to family, friends and loved ones. Special thanks to Dr Christine Page, MD and Drew Carter, and to Dr Trevor Cook for sharing his knowledge.

Thank you to my patients for trusting me to cherish their health.

The author and publishers would like to thank the following for the use of photographs in this volume:

p1 National Library of Medicine/Science Photo, **p2** Hulton Archive/Getty Images, **p3–4** Carl Drury, **p19** Winfried Wisniewski/FLPA, **p20** (left) **p35** (top) Inga Spence/Holt/FLPA, (right) Ainsworth Homeopathic Pharmacy, **p21, 23, 28** (top), **p30** (left), **p31, 32, 40, 44, 48, 49, 51, 52, 57, 64** GeoScience Features Picture Library, **p22** (left), **p36** Nigel Cattlin/Holt Studios/NHPA, **p24** © Tania Midgley/Corbis, **p25** © Lester V. Bergman/Corbis, **p26** © Buddy Mays/Corbis, **p27, 30** (right), **37, 39, 53, 55, 58** Bob Gibbons/Holt/FLPA, **p28** (top) Gordon Roberts/Holt/FLPA, **p33** Flip de Nooyer/Foto Natura/FLPA, **p34, 43** TH Foto-Werbung/Science Picture Library, **p37** (bottom), **p38** Charles D.Winters/Science Photo Library, **p41** © Klaus Hackenberg/ zefa/Corbis, **p42** dkimages.com, **p45** Michael and Patricia Fogden/ FLPA, **p46** Geoff Kidd/Science Photo Library, **p47** FLPA/David Hosking, **p50** P. Karanukaran/Holt/FLPA, **p54** M. Szadzuik/R.Zinck/FLPA, **p56** R.Dirscherl/FLPA, **p59, 62** Primrose Peacock/Holt/FLPA, **p60** E.R. Degginger/Science Photo Library, **p61** Roger Wilmshurst/ FLPA, **p63** Mike Amphlett/Holt/FLPA, **p141** © Royalty-Free, Corbis

contents

foreword

With the continuing growth in the practice of homeopathy worldwide, several useful introduction books are now available. It required, therefore, a book with special qualities to stand out from the others and *Homeopathy in Essence* by Andrew James can justifiably claim to satisfy the curiosity of the general public, those who wish to treat themselves or those who wish to find a sound launch-pad for more advanced studies to practitioner level.

As its title implies, this book presents the essence and subtlety of homeopathic practice and the natural remedies it employs in a logical, clearly understandable manner.

This book is a simple, direct presentation of the fundamental principles of homeopathy with helpful sketches of a number of homeopathic remedies used in the treatment of many day-to-day ailments. There are also guidelines on the theory of prescribing, where to obtain the remedies and where to learn more.

This book will provide a useful grounding for the newcomer. It deserves to succeed.

Trevor M. Cook, PhD, MSc, Dhom, DHM, MARH, FHMA, FRSC, FBIH
Director & Principal
The British Institute of Homeopathy
www.britinsthom.com

I trained in homeopathy in the late 1980s, having been brought up in a home where complementary medicine was the norm. During my medical training little time was given to such forms of health care, which I'm pleased to say is not the situation in today's medical schools. I remember the day when I realized that as a GP 80% of my patients were on permanent treatments for chronic illnesses and all I could say was, 'keep taking the tablets.' By offering homeopathy, I watched as not only did their symptoms diminish but 50% of those chronically ill patients were able to come off their treatments.

Despite claims of a mere placebo effect or lack of efficacy, millions of patients all over the world are grateful to their practitioners for their courage to move beyond skepticism and use what is one of the most holistic forms of energy medicine.

Homeopathy is not the easiest subject to understand, yet Andrew James has written an exciting and easy-to-read reference book for lay public and practitioners alike. His words move us effortlessly through the importance of recognizing homeopathy as complementary to mainstream medicine and towards a deeper appreciation of how a remedy with almost no material substance present, can bringing about such powerful healing effects.

Through his FAQ sections and helpful tips, he demystifies the modality, encouraging the reader to purchase and use homeopathic remedies as the first line of therapy for minor ailments or when faced with simple chronic complaints.

Andrew has always challenged himself to offer the most comprehensive and holistic approach to health care, whether in his practice or during his teaching. His generosity of spirit and enthusiasm for the subject exude from every page, making *Homeopathy in Essence* an essential book for any home or practitioner's library.

Dr. Christine Page, MD
Homeopath, lecturer and author of *Frontiers of Health*

Homeopathy is very much in the forefront of scientific debate regarding the evidence base supporting complementary medicine. There is a danger that this debate could hinder the progress of homeopathy, despite the fact that it is one of the most regulated fields of natural medicine. However, the popularity of homeopathy amongst the general public is growing despite criticism from some quarters of the scientific community. It is therefore inspiring to read a text book promoting professional practices, where homeopathy can be integrated with conventional medicine. This integrative approach is one I fully support. We should also recognise the fact that over the counter (OTC) homeopathic medicines are licensed by the Government Medicines and Healthcare products Regulatory Authority. This adds assurance of quality and safety to the OTC homeopathic medicines that Andrew recommends.

This book provides users of homeopathy with clear and concise information on how to self-treat common conditions. It is relevant for anyone who is searching for holistic treatments, which are able to resolve the emotional as well as physical conditions. It provides simple self-help remedies with examples of case histories where homeopathy has proved effective and highlights the indications which are often difficult to treat conventionally, such as in pregnancy. I believe that this book will serve as an effective introduction to anyone new to homeopathy as well as expanding the knowledge of those already converted!

By Kevin Leivers M.R.Pharm.S.
consultant for Weleda UK Ltd

Kevin Leivers is an independent consultant pharmacist with over 20 years experience in the conventional and natural pharmaceutical industry. For the last 10 years he has specialised in natural medicines including homeopathy. He has clients in the UK, USA, Australia, Germany and Scandinavia.

introduction

It was 1987 when I first started my journey into the world of 'complementary therapy'. At that time the therapies were more commonly known as 'alternative', which in some way implied that they were to replace conventional (allopathic) medicine. The very title 'alternative' was bound to arouse suspicion and criticism from the medical profession and it is easy to understand why this may have been the case.

At around this time I was asked to give a presentation to the staff of a large general practice on the subject, along with some other complementary or alternative therapists. To my horror the first speaker was telling parents how they could take their children off asthma drugs and replace them with nutritional changes and vitamin and mineral supplements. This speaker had no formal medical qualification and the doctors and nurses at the presentation were very upset, to say the least! I found this type of approach irresponsible and unprofessional. It was made worse by the appearance of the speaker, which was commented on by one of the doctors as 'all brown rice and sandals'. That comment has stayed with me to the present day, and I always stress to my students that a professional appearance and approach form a vital part of the image of a competent complementary practitioner.

When it came to my turn to speak I spent most of the time addressing the need for an integrated rather than alternative approach, and hopefully managed to salvage the reputation of complementary therapies in the minds of some of those present. I talked about how complementary therapies could assist with stress, pain relief, sleep problems and backache (to name but a few), and that the aim was to help the client, not to offer a cure. A cure could only be achieved by working with the client, alongside others who were responsible for the client's health, such as the medical profession. I also talked about the 'comfort and power of touch', which I believed was a vital part of therapies such as reflexology and massage, and how this was particularly relevant to those facing terminal illness, given that many complementary therapies have started to become part of patient care in hospitals and hospices. Indeed even as I write there have been several surveys relating to the care of the dying in hospital and hospices, where specialists working in the field say modern palliative care is changing the face of medicine, as it seeks to relieve the effects of illness rather than to cure the disease itself.

So from my earliest encounters with other alternative therapists and the medical profession I learnt that both sides needed to seek common ground and find respect for each other's strengths (and weaknesses) in order to achieve the best for patient care. I have now been working with complementary therapy for nearly two decades and there is certainly more integration and understanding of the role of complementary therapies, both within the world of complementary therapy and by the medical and other caring professions. This is due, in part, to better training, representation and governance of complementary therapies, but also to an improved understanding of their role by the medical profession, in their attempt to view patients more holistically.

With regard to homeopathy, in particular, the main criticism levelled against it by some of those in the scientific and medical professions is that there is no evidence that a particular remedy has any effect on the patient, and that any improvement to the client's condition can be attributed to the placebo effect. Those who support this view can point to any number of research papers and medical journals to strengthen their case; likewise, those who believe that the effect of homeopathy on the client is real, and is related to the dosage and type of remedy given, can also point to research materials to strengthen their case.

My own approach is to let the patient decide. There are many high street chemists and drugstores now selling homeopathic remedies. Recently I even observed arnica for sale in a petrol station, next to the paracetamol and aspirin! Although sales volumes do not prove the efficiency of the

remedies, it does give a strong indication that people want to buy them and that, by repeating this choice and becoming responsible for their own health, they affirm their effectiveness. The same arnica that was available in the petrol station is also being used in some hospital labour wards and care homes (a literal example of 'cradle to grave' care).

There are also many homeopathically qualified GPs and vets, adding validity to the theories and practice of homeopathy. My own GP recommended a patient to me who was suffering from IBS. The patient responded very well to homeopathic treatment and reported her findings back to the GP. In this way, patients themselves raise awareness of the benefits of homeopathic treatments, and further integration and acceptance will take place.

As a homeopath I recognize that there will always be a debate on the effectiveness of the treatment. The volumes of scientific research produced to date can be used to argue that the treatment cannot be proved to 'work' in the conventional sense, but this is by no means conclusive and much remains to be investigated. In the meantime it is the patient who is deriving benefit from the treatment and this is the area that requires our focus.

I believe that we have to be content in all areas of our lives to be truly whole (a tall order!). Homeopathy can really help a patient to understand themselves and their ailment. In my practice I want the client to use their knowledge and understanding of their own personality and how it interacts with their condition. By doing this we can reach the core of the homeopathic philosophy and truly prescribe a remedy that will allow them to move forward and help to create inner health. There is no such thing as a quick fix. Even conventional medicine cannot always offer such a tempting outcome (think of the surgeon replacing a hip joint – the patient still has to recover from the operation, learn to adapt and improve their posture in order to walk and then take responsibility for using it to improve their quality of life). So it is with any truly complementary therapy – the client sits at the centre of the process. In homeopathy we recognize this truth and concentrate on reaching an understanding of the core of the person. We may have to work through many layers to reach the core, but by doing so we can fully understand the effect of *their* ailment on *them*, and prescribe the remedy that is to reach their centre and do its work uniquely for them.

I also believe strongly that you do not have to be 'sick' in order for homeopathy to help with your health and well-being – start now! Develop an awareness of your overall state of health and use homeopathy to encourage and maintain your own uniqueness. I hope this book will encourage the understanding and use of homeopathic prescription and its unique approach to helping the patient.

Andrew James, D.I.HOM, FBIH, MAR, IFA
(Reg.), ITEC

what is homeopathy?

'**L**et like be cured with like'. The homeopathic principle is that when a substance is given to a healthy person they will show signs and symptoms in the form of the disease. If the substance is prepared homeopathically and given to a patient who is suffering with similar signs and symptoms, it is seen that health is restored through the rebalancing of energies.

How it began

Homeopathic theory began in 469–399 BC with the Greek physician Hippocrates. He believed that by observing the individual symptoms and reactions to a disease he could prescribe a remedy that would draw upon the patient's own powers of healing as well as the power of the remedy itself. This was in contrast to the conventional thinking of the time, which taught that the gods were the main force behind a disease and that a cure could be found by treatment with a substance that had an *opposite* effect in a healthy person – the complete reverse of the homeopathic principle.

The German doctor Samuel Hahnemann (1755–1843) was the modern-day founder of homeopathy. His experiments with quinine proved to him that 'like cures like'. Quinine was known to be an effective treatment for

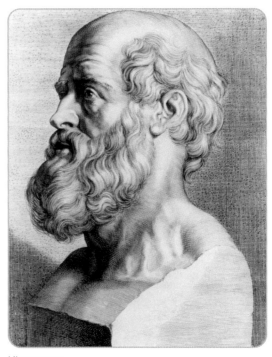

Hippocrates

malaria and so for several days he took doses of quinine. Although he was not suffering from malaria, after several doses of quinine he began to develop symptoms of the disease. The symptoms would begin after he had taken a dose of quinine and last for hours afterwards.

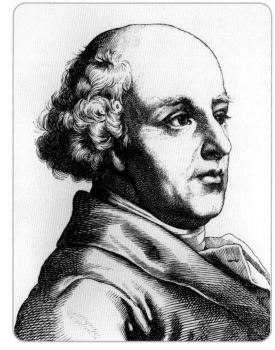

Samuel Hahnemann

To further develop his theory he began to test other substances used in medicine at the time in the same way. This time he used groups of volunteers. He recorded the effect of each substance on the individual, noting any reactions. This was called 'proving' the remedy. At the end of this process Hahnemann had listed many substances which could be used to treat a variety of conditions. It was important, however, to understand the nature of each person receiving the treatment, as he found that particular 'types' of people showed different symptoms for the same disease and therefore needed to be matched to the remedy closest to their type.

Hahnemann also believed the remedies acted on the person's 'vital force' (this is the body's own healing potential). He believed that the remedies helped to activate the body's vital force and trigger a reaction to fight a certain disease or condition. The type of remedy given would be the key to triggering the right reaction and stimulating the vital force to combat the disease or ailment. The remedy should therefore not only mirror the symptoms of the disease, but also the type of person taking the remedy. During his lifetime Hahnemann proved over a hundred homeopathic remedies. In 1811 he published *The Organon of Rationale Medicine*, which set out his theories and listed the many proved remedies.

American doctor James Tyler Kent (1849–1943) dedicated himself to homeopathy, continuing Hahnemann's work. He further developed the idea of types of people and that a remedy must be matched according to the emotional and physical characteristics of a person. These types became known as 'constitutional types'. He went on to write the *Kent Repertory*. The information in the repertory is stored under remedy headings, with emphasis given to mental and emotional symptoms.

Potentization – less is more!

Hahnemann believed in the vital force as a healing source and therefore wished to use the minimum amount of a substance to bring about the healing effect; this would also cause as few side effects as possible (known as aggravations). He discovered that if the substance was diluted it achieved a far better result. Thus the *less* the original substance remained in the remedy, the *greater* its potency. In order to get less of the original substance it must be diluted, so the greater the dilution, the more potent the remedy. This leads to the practice of potentization.

Remedies are potentized in the following way. An alcoholic/water extract is made from the material in question (called the mother tincture). The extract is then diluted to the required potency. The main potencies are: x = 1 in 10; c = 1 in 100; m = 1 in 1000. So a 1c potency is diluted 1 part mother tincture in 99 parts water. A 2c would take 1 part of the previous dilution and dilute again in 99 parts water and so on. The terms 'c', 'x' and 'm' therefore denote the degree of dilution of a particular remedy.

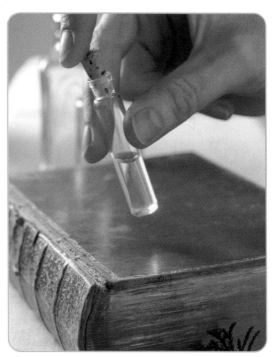

The original, clinical approach of succussion, tapping the vial on a book, is used by some homeopathic pharmacies. The main form of succussion is now performed by a machine.

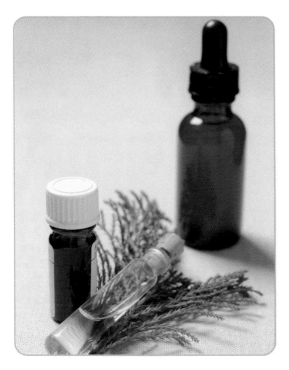

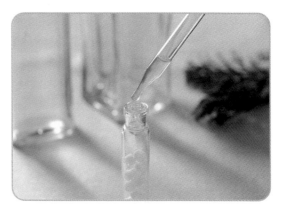

3

Before each dilution the mixture is shaken vigorously; this is known as succussion. Once the required potency is reached, a few drops of the substance are then applied to lactose (milk sugar) tablets and the tablets are placed in an airtight, dark-glass bottle and stored away from direct sunlight.

Sources of homeopathic remedies

A remedy can be made from virtually any source using the above method, but the most common sources are plants, trees, poisons and minerals.

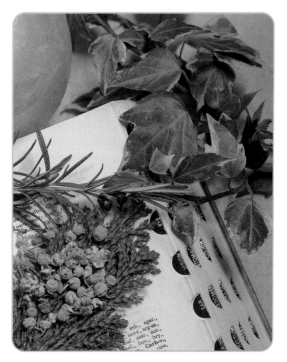

Modalities

Modalities are influences which worsen or improve the symptoms of the patient. They are an invaluable guide to the choice of a homeopathic remedy. Modalities can be in several forms, depending on the associated remedy:

- Physical modalities: movement, position of the body, touch, rest, exertion, noise and smells.

- Temperature modalities: hot, cold, warm, wind, season of the year, damp.

- Time modalities: day or night, morning, afternoon or evening; hourly (e.g. 10 a.m., 1 a.m., 3 p.m.).

- Dietary modalities: foods, drinks, stimulants, alcohol.

- Localized modalities: left-handed, right-handed, left worse, right worse.

The homeopathic aggravation

An 'aggravation' is the term given to a temporary worsening of the condition, which is viewed as a positive sign, meaning the remedy is working and has stimulated the vital force into the action of healing. For an acute condition the aggravation may last several hours; for a chronic case it may last up to two days. An improvement should follow after the aggravation. If an aggravation is experienced the remedy should be halted to allow the vital force and immune system to fight the condition. If the original symptom(s) begins to return the remedy should be taken again to provide further stimulation to the body's vital force.

Not everyone experiences an aggravation, and it is not necessary to experience one for the remedies to work; many people's conditions improve without an aggravation. If there is no improvement in the symptoms or condition, with or without an aggravation, this is an indication that a different remedy may be needed.

The vital force

This refers to the body's own subtle energy. The vital force may be run down by many factors, for example stress, poor diet and nutrition, hereditary conditions or lack of exercise. Homeopathic remedies stimulate the vital force to enable the body to heal itself by energizing it and enabling it to return to optimum health.

FAQs: Getting started

Is homeopathy safe?
I believe that the worst that can happen with homeopathic treatment is that the remedies do not work; that is to say, they do not achieve an effect. It is also prudent to state that homeopathic treatment is not a substitute for conventional medical treatment and that patients should always consult a doctor for treatment of any serious medical condition (although homeopathy can, of course, work alongside conventional medicines).

How many homeopathic remedies are there?
There are over 3000 remedies worldwide. This book covers the most used, useful and easily available remedies for common ailments. Further detailed study of remedies can be undertaken by reference to Boericke's *Materia Medica with Repertory*.

5

the homeopathic constitutions

Selecting a remedy can be based on the emotional and physical features of an individual as well as the illness or disease from which they are suffering. It is possible to identify several types of people for whom a particular remedy will be effective. A person may display many traits that fit into that particular type, irrespective of the disease or condition from which they are suffering. These types are known as 'constitutional types' and each is associated with a particular remedy.

Finding a constitutional type is rather like spotting the difference between a sports car and a van, and knowing that a sports car will run better on petrol while the van will need diesel fuel. Getting the right fuel for the right vehicle will improve the vehicle's performance. It does not, however, prevent individual engine trouble, for which the car may need 'super slick' spark plugs and the van may need 'super strong' engine oil. Thus a constitutional type may also need a different remedy on occasions, depending on the illness. Identifying the right combination is the trick!

When a person suffers from an ailment or illness, knowing their homeopathic constitution can be of great help in finding the remedy to treat the condition. Once this is achieved, the underlying causes of the illness can be treated as well as the symptoms, thus creating optimum health.

The homeopathic constitution is a whole picture of the individual, taking into account their physical, emotional and mental states. When selecting a remedy you should bear in mind mental and emotional factors and the constitutional type, as well as the presenting illness or disease.

Mental and emotional factors

The following factors should be taken into account when selecting remedies:

- ✿ The individual's fears and anxieties (e.g. fear of animals, spiders, the dark, thunderstorms, loneliness, robbery, attack, failure, death, poisoning).

- ✿ The individual's temperament – are they tearful, happy, sad, confident, lazy, perfectionist, mild, gentle, caring, optimistic, irritable, aggressive, spiteful?

- ✿ Whether certain things affect the individual on a personal level and whether they have an effect on the condition itself (e.g. Do they like noise around them? Does music bring on emotional reactions? Are they bright and alert in the morning or dull and unresponsive? Do they like their own company or prefer to be with others? Do they prefer hot or cold weather? Do they like dry or wet atmospheres? Do they talk to others about problems or keep themselves to themselves? Are there strong likes and dislikes for food and drinks? Are there cravings or intolerance to particular foods?)

Physical factors

The following factors should be taken into account when selecting remedies:

- ✿ Physical appearance. Are they tall or short? Fat or thin? Do they have long limbs? Are they underweight or overweight? Do they have dark rings under the eyes? What is their hair and eye colour? What sort of skin texture do they have? Is their skin tone even or uneven? Do they have a cracked lower lip? Do they have frown lines? Is their hair thick, curly, thin?

- ✿ Type of clothing. Is manner of dress formal or casual?

- ✿ Facial expressions. Do they look serious or have a relaxed look? Do they maintain eye contact or avoid it?

- ✿ Posture. Is it excellent? Do they slouch, constantly fidget, keep very still, keep their arms folded or crossed?

Since homeopathy was developed in Europe in the early nineteenth century, physical descriptions of the constitutional types reflect the society of that period rather than the multicultural societies of the present day. For that reason, you may have to pay more attention to emotional and mental aspects, but you can still take into account many of the physical factors, such as height, weight, build, long limbs, worried look, frown lines, dry, cracked lips, dark rings under the eyes, hair (curly, thick, thin, etc.), skin texture and shade, all of which can apply to any race or culture.

Constitutional types

Argent. Nit.

- **Physical appearance:** Pale complexion. Looks older than their years, due to worry and tension.

- **Mental/emotional aspects:** Often feels anxious. Always in a hurry to get somewhere or achieve something. Difficulty in controlling their emotions. Excellent at quick thinking and resolving problems. Can have an impulsive streak and a tendency to be an extrovert to hide true feelings.

- **Physical weakness:** Nervous system. Digestive system. Eyes. Ailments tend to be more on the left side of the body.

- **Food likes/dislikes:** Likes and craves chocolates and sweets, salt and cheese. Dislikes chilled/cold foods.

- **Child:** Always moving around and never wants to sit still. Prone to upset stomachs or nerves when stressed. Will react badly to new situations that are unhappy (e.g. changing school). Can become prone to bed-wetting.

Arsen. Alb.

- **Physical appearance:** Usually thin or slim. Often well groomed and stylish. Fine facial features, with delicate, sensitive skin. Frown lines can appear on the forehead.

- **Mental/emotional aspects:** Restless individuals. Perfectionists at work and at home. Can be critical and intolerant. Strongly opinionated. Can have a deep fear of being alone. Obsessive compulsive behaviour, in particular involving cleanliness and tidying up – this can hide a hoarding mentality! Can pull out of plans and projects early if they think it is not going to work out 100 per cent. Pessimistic in nature, with a need to receive constant reassurance.

- **Physical weakness:** Digestive system. Skin. Respiratory system (asthma, coughs and colds).

- **Food likes/dislikes:** Likes fatty foods, warm food and drinks, in particular coffee, sweets, alcohol and sour-tasting foods. Dislikes large amount of fluid.

- **Child:** Extremely sensitive and highly strung. Upsets easily with loud noise. Becomes tired and exhausted quickly after periods of exertion. Suffers nightmares due to very active imagination. Increasingly physically and mentally agile with age. Can worry too much about parents' health and well-being. Keeps room neat and tidy. Does not like mess or getting messy (avoids paint, mud, etc.).

Calc. Carb.

- **Physical appearance:** Overweight or gains weight easily. Possesses a large appetite. Sluggish, bloated and tired in appearance. May have poor posture. Can be hardy despite weight.

- **Mental/emotional aspects:** Impressionable. Sensitive and quiet. May have a deep fear of failure that can make them withdrawn. Can dwell on and worry too much about a particular problem and begin to fixate. Cruelty to children and animals upsets them greatly.

Needs motivation to succeed in tasks. Can be prone to mild depression when unwell; reassurance from loved ones results in immediate improvement of condition.

- **Physical weakness:** ears, nose and throat. Skeletal system (e.g. backache). Skin. Teeth. Chronic fatigue syndrome. Exhaustion. TATT (tired all the time). Depression. Digestive disorders, in particular IBS (irritable bowel syndrome) and feelings of bloatedness.

- **Food likes/dislikes:** Likes dairy and egg products, sweets, salt, desserts of any nature, chocolate, carbohydrates, cool/ice drinks and ice cream. Dislikes fatty meat, boiled food and milk.

- **Child:** Plump and overweight. Often skin and complexion is pale. Slow to walk and talk. Can fall over easily in the early stages of walking. Lazy and scared of the dark. Prone to nightmares. Needs encouragement with schoolwork.

Graphites

- **Physical appearance:** Rough, dry skin. Dry hair, which is usually dark in colour. Skin can be cracked and flake easily. Prone to being overweight. Blushes easily. Can have a rugged, windswept appearance. Flaky scalp. Large appetite.

- **Mental/emotional aspects:** A 'plodder' – takes time to work things out and arrive at a solution. Deep concentration on a task can make them irritable. Prone to mood swings. Unwilling to change attitudes and routines. Not at their best first thing in the morning. Can become tearful and despondent, followed by impatience.

- **Physical weakness:** All skin problems. Soreness in the corners of the mouth. Slow metabolic rate. Exhaustion. Nail problems. Obesity. Bad breath. Nosebleeds. Styes. Travel sickness.

- **Food likes/dislikes:** Likes sour and savoury foods and cool drinks. Dislikes sweet foods, seafood and shellfish, salt and hot drinks.

- **Child:** Feels the cold and becomes chilly very quickly. Timid and hesitant, leading to anxiousness. Does not like long periods of travel, which can lead to sickness.

Ignatia

- **Physical appearance:** Most often used as a woman's constitutional remedy, although some men may fall into this as well. Dark to medium hair, and a slim build. Prone to dark circles under the eyes and may have involuntary twitching of the eyes and mouth. Often have dry lips, with a tired, drawn expression. Sighs a lot.

- **Mental/emotional aspects:** Out of all the constitutional types Ignatia is the most highly strung, with a tendency to rapid and extreme mood swings. Can switch quickly from depression to joy and from tears to laughter. Prone to suppressing grief and finds it difficult to end relationships. May punish themselves for not having the strength to end relationships and may develop grief for themselves for not being stronger. There is a tendency to develop fixed ideas about their health, which can lead to hypochondria and, in extreme cases, obsessive compulsive disorder. Addictions to tobacco and coffee are also likely.

- **Physical weakness:** Nervous system. Hysterical grief over bereavement, leading to depression, twitching and grinding of teeth. Headaches. Sore throats, coughs and colds. Constipation. Emotional trauma may be the cause of any number of physical problems.

- **Food likes/dislikes:** Likes sour and savoury foods, dairy products and carbohydrates. Likes coffee, but may not always agree with them. Dislikes sweet foods.

- **Child:** Highly strung. Very excitable, yet sensitive. Finds it difficult to perform under stress. Finds separation/divorce of parents very hard to deal with, leading to outbursts of anger, crying and performing less well at school. Prefers company to being alone. May suffer with headaches, coughs and sore throats. Responds well to reassurance.

Lachesis

- **Physical appearance:** Strong and fixed expression. Strong and staring eyes. Wears loose clothing around the neck (hates restrictive clothes in this area). Hair colour is often light to medium. Prone to slight freckles. May have a bloated look, but can also be lean in the body. Complexion is usually pale. Can lick the lips a lot.

- **Mental/emotional aspects:** Very ambitious. Highly creative. Can become crowded in thought and allow too many distractions. Jealousy is their worst trait, which can lead to loved ones and friends being driven away. Highly talkative, particularly about themselves. Possessive of friends and family. Hates tight clothing

as it makes them feel constricted around the throat and waist. Can be sensitive to noise, which leads to stress. If religious, then prone to view themselves as sinful. Not good first thing in the morning. Can be very suspicious of others and new introductions. Can be their own worst enemy.

- **Physical weakness:** All circulatory problems (e.g. varicose veins). Nervous system. Hyperactivity. Menopausal problems. Sore throats and asthma. Disturbed sleep and insomnia. Palpitations and panic attacks. Prone to left-sided problems. Physical problems made worse when trying to sleep or remain still.

- **Food likes/dislikes:** Likes coffee, alcohol, seafood, cool drinks, sour and savoury food and carbohydrates. Dislikes sweet drinks.

- **Child:** Attention deficit disorder. Spiteful and possessive. Hyperactive. Jealous of siblings, particularly newborns. Nightmares.

Lycopodium

- **Physical appearance:** Tall, with a lean look. Worry and frown lines on the forehead. Thinning hair in men. Facial twitches. Can look older than their years.

- **Mental/emotional aspects:** Prone to exaggeration. Can create a drama over minor matters. Insecure and hates any form of change. Avoids commitment. Always becomes anxious of forthcoming challenges. Strong fear of being alone and of the dark. Forgetful. Small mistakes can irritate them disproportionately. Hates contradiction.

- **Physical weakness:** Chronic fatigue syndrome. Headaches. Sore throats. All digestive problems. Kidney stones. Prostate problems. Male pattern baldness. Alopecia. Dislikes tight clothing. Right-sided problems are more prevalent.

- **Food likes/dislikes:** Likes sweet foods, warm drinks, onions, garlic, fish and shellfish, desserts, cakes and biscuits. Dislikes cheese and strong-flavoured meats.

- **Child:** Insecure and shy. Likes to be indoors. Likes to read and is good academically. Can be bossy and dominant with other children.

Merc. Sol.

- **Physical appearance:** Skin on the face may be shiny or moist due to perspiration, with a grey, translucent look. The hair may be fair to medium. The body is of medium build. Often they have a look of relaxed detachment.

- **Mental/emotional aspects:** May have an inner battle with their emotions. Resentment, anxiety and lack of trust in others may lead to deep feelings of insecurity. They do not like criticism or taking orders from others. They may explode with rage and anger. Their memory may become poor with age and thought patterns may become detached later in life.

- **Physical weakness:** Sore throats. Swelling of glands. Chronic fatigue syndrome. Exhaustion. TATT (tired all the time). Mouth ulcers and gum problems. Bad breath. Cold sores. Tired and aching limbs. Very sensitive to changes in the weather

and may suffer from SAD (seasonal affective disorder). Conjunctivitis. Skin sensitivity and allergies.

- **Food likes/dislikes:** Likes cold drinks, carbohydrates, zesty and citrus fruits. Dislikes strong-flavoured meats, sweet, rich foods and salt.

- **Child:** Irritating, precocious behaviour when in surroundings that encourage confidence, such as with family and friends. Can be shy and cautious outside the family. May have a tendency to stammer. Weakness in the ear and susceptible to ear, nose and throat ailments. Irritable when unwell.

Nat. Mur.

- **Physical appearance:** Pear-shaped build in women. Solid, strong to lean build in men. Skin can be oily and puffy, with a tendency to swell. Redness around the eyes, which may also be watery in appearance. Lips can look dry and cracked, particularly on the lower lip. Medium to dark hair.

- **Mental/emotional aspects:** Prone to suppressing emotions such as fear, loneliness, guilt and anger, which can lead to depression. Feelings of grief or loss for a loved one or for the self that are never shaken off or are suppressed for many years before coming to the surface. Career-minded and successful, with a serious outlook on life. With a marriage or relationship break-up they can become very despondent and depressed. May want to cry but cannot. Other people do not realize how sensitive the Nat. Mur. type is. They are prone to suffer in silence and not ask for help when it is needed.

- **Physical weakness:** Nervous system, triggered by unresolved loss and grief. Depression. Premenstrual syndrome. Anorexia. Skin problems. Mouth ulcers and cold sores. Palpitations. Headaches. Craving for salt.

- **Food likes/dislikes:** Likes salt, cool drinks, sour and savoury foods and craves most carbohydrates. Dislikes coffee and bread.

- **Child:** May be small for their age. Slow physical and mental development. Well behaved and integrates well with other children and adults. Loves animals and looks after them well. Excellent at school, but if criticized at school can become very hurt. Can be prone to headaches under pressure.

Nux Vomica

- **Physical appearance:** More often a male type. Looks stressed and tense and has a slim or lean appearance, particularly when young. Prone to dark circles under the eyes. Ages prematurely. Smart appearance. Face can become red and flushed, through anger or excitement.

- **Mental/emotional aspects:** Can suffer from addictions and overindulgence. May have cravings for alcohol, food and stimulants such as coffee and cigarettes. Can be addicted to sex. Finds it difficult to relax and switch off. Can be very ambitious, often at the expense of others. Impatient. Intolerant and critical as they often require perfection in others. Whatever is done for a Nux Vomica type, they will always find fault with it. The worst thing that can happen to a Nux Vomica type is failure.

- **Physical weakness:** Digestive system. Migraines and headaches. Hernia. Indigestion and heartburn from hangovers and overindulgence. Hay fever. Feels better for sleep.

- **Food likes/dislikes:** Likes fatty and rich foods, cheese and cream, alcohol, coffee and spicy foods. Dislikes the effect of some strongly spiced food (although likes to eat it!).

- **Child:** Irritable. Can become bored easily, leading to hyperactivity or ADD (attention deficit disorder). Can throw tantrums easily. Becomes competitive as a teenager and cannot bear to lose. When upset or stressed it can show in stomach pains and disorders. Can become addicted to alcohol and drugs in teenage years. Likes to be the rebel.

Phosphorus

- **Physical appearance:** Tall and slim, with long limbs. Can have fair to dark hair. Fine skin. Likes to dress well and look stylish. Can be artistic and creative in appearance.

- **Mental/emotional aspects:** Needs a lot of love and attention. Good fun to be with, but can be very needy and demanding. Likes to be the centre of attention. Enjoys sympathy when upset or unwell. Finds it easy to be expressive and affectionate. Shows emotions easily. Needs reassurance, in particular with looks and body image. Short attention span. Challenging, particularly towards a wife or partner.

- **Physical weakness:** Circulation problems. Nervous system – in particular fear and hypersensitivity. Vertigo. Coughs and colds. Weakness of the lungs. Headaches. Prone to left-sided problems.

🖘 **Food likes/dislikes:** Likes salt, spicy food, sour and savoury food, carbonated drinks, alcohol (wine, in particular), mild cheeses and sweet foods. Dislikes strong-flavoured fish and fruit.

🖘 **Child:** Tall and slim, with long legs and arms. Nervous. Likes to be surrounded by people. Likes to be the centre of attention. Loves to receive affection – cuddles, in particular. Has a strong fear of the dark.

Pulsatilla

🖘 **Physical appearance:** Mainly a female type. A gentle and kind appearance. Shy in nature. Hair is fair and skin has a rosy complexion. Usually has blue eyes. Can be slightly overweight. Blushes easily. A young appearance despite their age. Often rests with hands behind the head.

🖘 **Mental/emotional aspects:** Kind and gentle, but likes to be supported by others. Makes friends easily. Becomes embarrassed easily. Not easily assertive and can be very indecisive. Cries and weeps easily, in particular over cruelty to children and animals, tragic news or weepy movies. Laughs easily. Avoids confrontation. Loves animals and animals love them. Acts on their emotions. Can suppress guilt and anger. Occasionally prone to obsessive or compulsive behaviour.

🖘 **Physical weakness:** All female reproductive problems. Catarrh. IBS (irritable bowel syndrome). Skin problems. Varicose veins. Styes. Physical symptoms can fluctuate and change rapidly.

🖘 **Food likes/dislikes:** Likes sweet foods, chocolates and cakes, cold foods and cool drinks. Dislikes fatty foods, very rich, spicy food and cream or butter.

🖘 **Child:** Dislikes bedtime. Fear of the dark. Sensitive to changes in the weather. Becomes tearful and weepy when overtired. Prone to coughs and colds.

Sepia

🖘 **Physical appearance:** Mainly a female type, but can apply to some men. Slim and tall. Medium to dark hair, often with brown eyes. Often sits with legs crossed. Likes to look attractive and elegant.

🖘 **Mental/emotional aspects:** Can be irritable and easily offended. Tendency to be aggressive to loved ones. Cannot handle too much stress. Tries to escape pressure and deadlines. Weeping makes them feel better, but dislikes people fussing around them. Avoids crowds. Hates contradiction as they always hold strong opinions. Deep fear of being alone.

🖘 **Physical weakness:** All menopausal problems. Headaches and migraine. Skin problems. Constipation and haemorrhoids. Chronic fatigue syndrome. Depression. Left-sided problems. Conditions usually improve with exertion.

🖘 **Food likes/dislikes:** Likes spices, sour and savoury food, citrus fruits, sweets and sweet foods and alcohol. Dislikes dairy products (in particular, milk). Also dislikes rich, strong-flavoured meats and fatty foods.

🖘 **Child:** Greedy with food. Prone to constipation. Can become a bed-wetter. Moody. Feels the cold and becomes tired easily. Does not like being alone.

Silicea

🔹 **Physical appearance:** Often slim or thin-looking, with large forehead. The head can appear too large for the body, but with delicate, fine features – almost doll-like in appearance. The hair may look thin or fine, but tidy in appearance. The skin of the lips looks grey and can be cracked. The palms of the hand feel sweaty to touch and the nails can be brittle.

🔹 **Mental/emotional aspects:** Appears to have low confidence from a young age. Prone to mental exhaustion. Can become overburdened, overwhelmed. Responsibility weighs heavily upon the Silicea type. They can be indecisive when deciding to take on new tasks or projects, in particular with house moves and new jobs. When a decision is made they can then develop into workaholics, owing to their strong fear of failure. Fear of failure can also spread into their relationships. When given advice from loved ones and close friends they can reply with a stubborn attitude in order to hide their true feelings. They can become very nervous about special events, such as interviews, presentations and performances.

🔹 **Physical weakness:** Nervous system, in particular burnout from new ventures. Exhaustion. Slowness in healing and convalescence. Respiratory illnesses and weaknesses. Chest infections. Low resistance to coughs and colds. Constipation. Skin problems. Headaches. Feels the cold.

🔹 **Food likes/dislikes:** Likes cold food, such as salads and raw vegetables. Dislikes meat and dairy products, in particular cheese and milk. Also dislikes food served very hot.

🔹 **Child:** Can look small for their age, with a petite appearance, apart from the head, which may look large for the body size. Always feels chilly and cold before everyone else. Feels the need to wrap up well, in particular to keep the head warm. Not the best child with sports activities as they may lack stamina and be shy. Usually tidy and well-behaved.

Sulphur

🔹 **Physical appearance:** Varied in appearance. Hair can be coarse and dry and look untidy. May have a slightly untidy appearance, as if just out of bed. Often looks happy and cheerful. Skin can be prone to redness, in particular the lips. May be slim and lean, with poor posture.

🔹 **Mental/emotional aspects:** Mind and house can be cluttered. Can be critical, even over the smallest matter. Prone to being selfish and self-centred. Likes to argue and enjoys debate and discussion. Can be generous and open-hearted. May lack will-power and self-esteem, which can hold back relationships and careers. Can move too quickly between projects and ideas, without seeing them through to the end.

🔹 **Physical weakness:** Skin problems. Weakness in the circulation. Haemorrhoids and constipation. Hot, burning feet. Body odour. Dislike of washing.

🐾 **Food likes/dislikes:** Likes sweet foods, fatty foods and stimulants such as coffee and chocolate. Likes alcohol, spicy foods, savoury foods, citrus fruits and seafood. Dislikes dairy, in particular milk and eggs. Dislikes most hot drinks.

🐾 **Child:** Untidy-looking. Can become hyperactive in the evening and does not like going to bed. Does not like bathing, showers or hand-washing. Has a very healthy appetite.

Recognizing constitutional types

Another way of thinking about constitutional types is to imagine yourself at a large family gathering: look round the room and use your observational skills to try to recognize some of the constitutions you might encounter. For example:

🐾 Person looks tense and older than their years: **Argent. Nit.**

🐾 Person is sensitive, has a large appetite, sluggish nature and poor posture: **Calc. Carb.**

🐾 Person has dark circles under their eyes, is highly strung, with mood swings and a tendency towards depression: **Ignatia.**

🐾 Person has strong, staring eyes, is prone to possessiveness and jealousy, and is creative and ambitious: **Lachesis.**

Using constitutional types

By learning to work with the constitution, true healing begins to take place. By treating the individual's overall profile, we are able to reach the heart and soul of the patient, finding a perfect remedy match to stimulate their vital force. Using the information about constitutional types (above), the following example demonstrates how an individual's type will help to identify the best remedy.

A person is suffering from a sore throat and cold.

🐾 The best remedy that fits this individual's *own* physical symptoms relating to a sore throat and cold is either Aconite, Silicea or Gelsemium (see Chapter 3: The remedies).

🐾 The best remedy for this individual's *own* emotional aspects (which may or may not be connected directly to a sore throat and cold) is either Silicea or Gelsemium (see Chapter 3: The remedies).

🐾 The best remedy according to this individual's *own* constitution is Silicea (taken from the 'Constitutional types' section, above).

🐾 Select Silicea.

It is not essential to calculate the remedy in this way – prescribing Aconite or Gelsemium based on the physical symptoms only *will* have an effect – but the *best effect* would be Silicea, as it fits all aspects for that individual.

casestudy: Female, 25 years

A woman came to me, via the local GP, for treatment of IBS. During the initial consultation I established that her discomfort was on the right side of the bowel area. She also had regular feelings of bloating, even after small meals. These symptoms were worse in the late afternoon and early evening. She reported feeling the cold easily. In my opinion she also looked a little older than her years. She confessed to losing a lot of her self-confidence, as the IBS had created problems with flatulence, which had caused her embarrassment on more than one occasion. She was employed in a job that required a great deal of intellect. She further reported restless legs while sleeping on several occasions since the onset of the IBS – this had disturbed her sleep and she had begun to feel extremely tired during the day.

This patient exhibited many of the indicators for the remedy Lycopodium, especially on a constitutional level. Her modalities matched the pattern of worse for heat and overeating and better for movement. Her likes and dislikes also matched with Lycopodium – she liked sweet foods and warm drinks and disliked meat (she was a non-meat eater), although she ate fish (but not seafood). I prescribed Lycopodium, 30c three times a day for three days, then twice a day for two to three days, then ceasing for two days until she saw me again.

At our next appointment the IBS had subsided significantly and she reported only a tense feeling in her stomach, but no discomfort. She did admit to still feeling very stressed, however. I decided to prescribe Kali Phos. (known as the great nerve soother), one to be taken for five to seven days, then one every other day for five days, and then to return for a further appointment. When I next saw her she reported no reoccurrence of the IBS. She also reported an amazing reduction in her stress levels, which in turn had made her feel less exhausted. I did have in mind a further prescription of Zinc. Met. to help with the restless legs if she was still feeling exhausted, but as she had made such good progress I felt this was not necessary.

FAQs: Constitutional types

Why the constitutional treatment?
The treatment is holistic and takes into account the physical condition, the emotional aspect and the mental state. In this way the mind, body and spirit are linked to give an overall effective treatment.

I fall into more than one constitution – how do I choose the right one?
Try the one closest to your personality by matching your likes, dislikes and health condition (mental and emotional aspects) with those of the remedy. If you improve, but feel there are still some aspects of your condition that have not fully recovered, select a further remedy based on the changed condition and your reaction to it. In other words, your constitutional aspect will vary according to the progress of the treatment and your own circumstances at a particular time – this is when a new remedy may help.

Each person's constitution can fall across several types; therefore it may be that the first strongly matched remedy does not create the right effect, and a further remedy, which is also indicated, may achieve better results. This can be common when an individual's personality traits are complex.

I am of African descent and wonder, given that the constitutional types outlined seem to refer mainly to European physical characteristics (blue eyes, pale skin, etc.), how I determine my own type?
Skin and eye colour are only part of the overall physical characteristics. Other physical indicators, such as height, weight, long limbs, frown lines, strong, staring eyes, older- or younger-looking for their years, and so on, are applicable to all races. Indeed skin colour in terms of paler or darker can also be applicable to those of African descent. Bear this in mind along with identifying your strong mental and emotional characteristics and it is possible to determine your type.

Do you always treat a person with the remedy that matches their constitutional type?
Yes and no! Yes, if you are trying to treat a deep-rooted condition, whether emotional or physical, as this will be more effective at reaching a deeper healing level. No, if the condition is acute (e.g. a sudden headache, exam nerves, anxiety before an appointment, etc.), as the remedy is to target the immediate symptoms and condition.

the remedies

Aconite

Derived from: monkshood, a toxic plant used for centuries to treat infections and also as a poison arrow in hunting.

Useful to treat when any of the following **mental/emotional aspects** are indicated:

- Anxiety and great fear.
- Feelings of doom and gloom, especially when accompanied by illness.
- A strong fear of death, the dark and ghosts.
- Agoraphobia and panic.
- Any form of shock.
- Worry and stress about the future.
- Nightmares.
- Panic attacks.
- Vivid imagination.
- Unhappiness.
- Emotional and physical tension that creates a draining of energy from the mind and body.

Useful to treat when any of the following **physical aspects** are indicated:

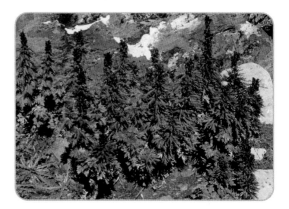

- Headaches, with a hot and heavy sensation.
- Red, inflamed eyes, with a feeling of grittiness.
- Ear problems, especially if hot, painful and swollen.
- Throbbing nose.

- ❧ Sore throat that feels dry and constricted.
- ❧ Tightness and pressure around the chest area.
- ❧ Palpitations.
- ❧ Coughs, colds and influenza.
- ❧ Sunburn, when accompanied by shaking and fever.
- ❧ Sleep problems, in particular waking in the night or difficulty falling asleep.
- ❧ Feelings of restlessness when trying to relax.
- ❧ Twitching of the eye when nervous.
- ❧ Any illness with a sudden onset.

Modalities

Better: for fresh air and warmth.
Worse: in the evening and at night.

Treatment tips

When treating with Aconite, always think 'sudden onset', such as fevers, colds, pain and inflammation that arrive suddenly.

It is suggested that you add this remedy to your homeopathic first aid kit.

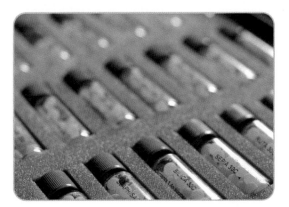

A homeopathic first aid kit

Allium

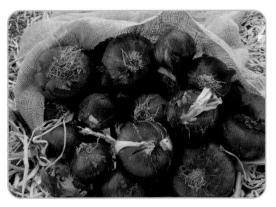

Derived from: fresh red onions. Grown since ancient times in China, India and the Middle East for its healing potential.

Useful to treat when any of the following **mental/emotional aspects** are indicated:

- ❧ Fear of pain.

Useful to treat when any of the following **physical aspects** are indicated:

- ❧ Headaches, with a head cold.
- ❧ Headaches emanating from the forehead.
- ❧ Streaming eyes and nose.
- ❧ Coughs and colds.
- ❧ Nasal discharge, with sneezing and coughing.
- ❧ Earache in children.

- ◊ Sore nostrils.
- ◊ Blocked nose.
- ◊ Catarrh.
- ◊ Watery and sore eyes.
- ◊ Hoarse throat and tickling throat with cough.
- ◊ Hay fever.
- ◊ Swollen eyes.
- ◊ Conjunctivitis.

Modalities

Better: for cool and damp atmosphere; fresh air.
Worse: in warm rooms; in the evening; when cold and damp; with pollen and around flowers.

Treatment tips

Excellent remedy of choice when there are symptoms of streaming eyes and nose, along with soreness and swelling.

Alumina

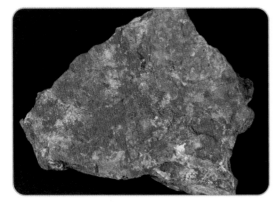

Derived from: aluminium oxide. The remedy is made from the rock bauxite, which is composed of hydrated aluminium oxide.

Useful to treat when any of the following **mental/emotional aspects** are indicated:

- ◊ Depression.
- ◊ Memory loss.
- ◊ Eating disorders (anorexia).
- ◊ Poor concentration.
- ◊ Apprehension.
- ◊ Negative outlook.

- ◊ Sensitivity to sharp objects.
- ◊ Sluggish attitude.
- ◊ Mood swings.
- ◊ Despair.
- ◊ SAD (seasonal affective disorder).
- ◊ TATT (tired all the time).
- ◊ Emotional and physical tension that creates a draining of energy from the mind and body.

Useful to treat when any of the following **physical aspects** are indicated:

- ◊ Loss of appetite.
- ◊ Headaches and dizziness.
- ◊ Weak and numb limbs.
- ◊ Fatigue.
- ◊ Chronic fatigue syndrome.
- ◊ Constipation.
- ◊ Hard, dry stools.
- ◊ Much straining to pass a stool.
- ◊ Sluggish bowels, can be changeable – better one day and worse the next.

Modalities

Better: for fresh air and summer weather.
Worse: in the morning; eating; during winter.

Treatment tips

A good remedy to use against the toxic effect of aluminium. Also excellent for constipation.

Apis Mel.

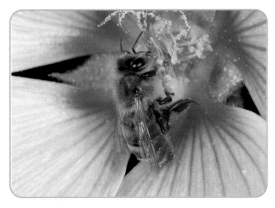

Derived from: the honeybee. The whole bee is used for this remedy; thus it is very useful for treating stinging conditions. Propolis, a resin-type substance used by the bee to seal up holes in the hive, has been used for centuries as a natural antibiotic.

Useful to treat when any of the following **mental/emotional aspects** are indicated:

- Poor memory.
- Feelings of jealousy.
- Hard to please.
- Tearfulness.
- Apathy and indifference.

Useful to treat when any of the following **physical aspects** are indicated:

- Clumsiness.
- Headaches, with a stabbing and stinging pain.
- All eye problems that sting and burn.

- Itchy, stinging skin.
- Arthritis, when the pain is burning in sensation.
- Cystitis and other urinary tract infections that cause stinging on passing urine.
- Insect bites and stings.
- Skin that is sensitive to touch.
- A constant, spasmodic cough.

Modalities

Better: for cool water and a cool room; the application of cold compresses.
Worse: for pressure and touch; heat.

Treatment tips

An excellent remedy for swollen and itchy skin, particularly insect bites and stings.

It is suggested that you add this remedy to your homeopathic first aid kit.

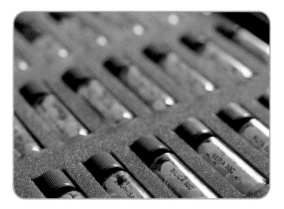

Argent. Nit.

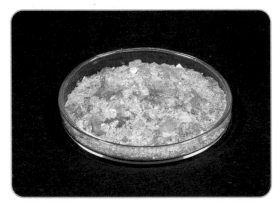

Derived from: silver nitrate (a compound of silver). Poisonous in large amounts. Was used to cauterize wounds, due to its caustic nature.

Useful to treat when any of the following **mental/emotional aspects** are indicated:

- Apprehension.
- Fearfulness.
- Nervousness.
- Overactive imagination.
- Stage fright.
- Phobias, in particular claustrophobia and fear of spiders and insects.
- Always feeling stressed and in a hurry.
- Constant worry.
- Fear of giving talks or addressing groups.
- Fear of exams.

Useful to treat when any of the following **physical aspects** are indicated:

- Diarrhoea caused by anxiety and tension.
- Tight, sore muscles through constant body tension.
- Headaches brought about by periods of concentration.
- Flatulence.
- Trembling and weakness in muscles and limbs.
- Palpitations and tightness of the chest.
- Nightmares.
- Aching, tired eyes.
- IBS (irritable bowel syndrome).

Modalities

Better: for cool, fresh air and pressure.
Worse: for concentration; when highly emotional; warmth.

Treatment tips

A remedy which helps combat apprehension and anxiety. Useful when there is fear of a known event, for example an exam or interview. Helps with the event itself, but also helps to combat the worry and stress leading up to the event.

Arnica

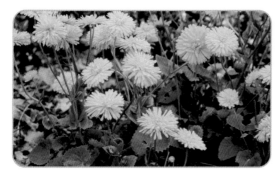

Derived from: leopard's bane, a plant used since the sixteenth century as a remedy for bruises, muscular aches and pains and rheumatism.

Useful to treat when any of the following **mental/emotional aspects** are indicated:

- Irritability.
- Nervousness.
- Inability to stay focused on a task.
- Forgetful and indifferent.
- Agoraphobia.
- All forms of shock.
- Bereavement.
- Oversensitivity.

Useful to treat when any of the following **physical aspects** are indicated:

- Following all forms of surgery, including dental.
- Swelling.
- Bruising.
- Labour pains and childbirth.
- Sore muscles.
- Backache and joint pain.
- Sprains.
- Black eyes.

- Accidents and falls.
- Hot, sensitive, aching headache.
- Heavy, tired eyes.
- Concussion.
- Nosebleeds.
- Sore muscles in chest following a bad cough.
- Overexertion due to exercise, gardening, and so on.
- Vertigo.

Modalities

Better: for lying down.
Worse: for continued movement; cold, damp weather.

Treatment tips

Arnica is a key remedy for all forms of muscular pain and bruising. It is also very useful applied topically to unbroken skin in a cream or ointment form, or as a compress using the tincture. Arnica is one of the most commonly used remedies and is a best-seller over the counter.

It is suggested that you add this remedy to your homeopathic first aid kit.

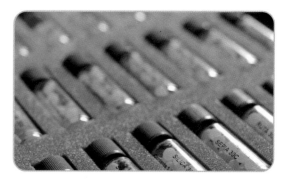

Arsen. Alb.

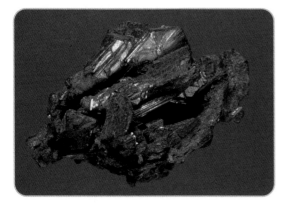

Derived from: arsenic, the mineral, which is a metallic poison.

Useful to treat when any of the following **mental/emotional aspects** are indicated:

- Great restlessness.
- Anguish and anxiety.
- Feelings of hopelessness.
- Possible overreaction to ailments and conditions.
- Agitation.
- Hypochondria.
- Perfectionism, demonstrated by obsessive compulsive behaviour.
- Inability to cope.
- Insecurity.
- Fear of the dark.
- Fear of poisoning.
- Twitches.
- Fixed ideas.
- Jealousy.

- Addictions, such as alcohol and tobacco.
- Fear of being alone.
- Fear of death.
- Fear of suffocation.

Useful to treat when any of the following **physical aspects** are indicated:

- Skin, hair and scalp problems, such as psoriasis and dandruff.
- Food poisoning.
- Vomiting.
- Exhaustion or TATT (tired all the time).
- Headaches.
- Mouth ulcers.
- Fluid retention.
- Mild forms of asthma.
- Sore throat, particularly if swallowing is difficult.
- Cramp.
- Disturbed, restless sleep.
- Angina pain.

Modalities

Better: for warm drinks; heat and movement.
Worse: for cold and wet weather.

Treatment tips

A very useful remedy for the treatment of digestive problems. Also excellent for treating anxiety and restlessness. Acts on every organ and tissue of the body.

Aurum Met.

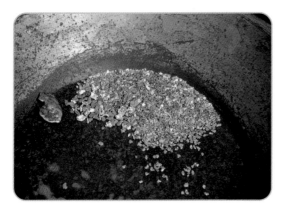

Derived from: the precious metal gold, ground to a powder.

Useful to treat when any of the following **mental/emotional aspects** are indicated:

- Tendency to become a workaholic.
- Setting very high standards for themselves, which often are impossible to live up to and drive those surrounding them to distraction.
- Prone to perfectionism, leading to dissatisfaction with their own achievements.
- Can become deeply upset and hurt if criticized.
- Extreme unhappiness.
- Depression, sometimes leading to suicidal thoughts.
- Grief can trigger illness.
- Fixed ideas.
- Can become obsessed with illness and death.
- Prone to criticize everyone around them.
- Cannot always share their inner worries with others, but will brood internally on problems.
- Nightmares.
- Loud noise can bring on anxiety.

Useful to treat when any of the following **physical aspects** are indicated:

- Illness through depression.
- Heart disease, blood and circulatory problems.
- Headaches.
- Chest pain and feelings of breathlessness.
- Sinus problems and sinusitis.
- Catarrh.
- Ear, nose and throat problems.
- Joint pain and skin ulcers.
- SAD (seasonal affective disorder).

Modalities

Better: for fresh air and movement.
Worse: emotional stress and tension; at night; in wintertime.

Treatment tips

A good remedy to try when others have failed, in particular for depression where there appears to be no 'light at the end of the tunnel'.

Belladonna

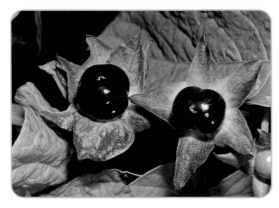

Derived from: the deadly nightshade plant. Popular during the middle ages for magic rituals. One of the first homeopathic remedies used to treat scarlet fever.

Useful to treat when any of the following **mental/emotional aspects** are indicated:

- Sudden anger.
- Feelings of guilt.
- Stress.
- Depression triggered by agitation.
- Sudden temper tantrums, accompanied by redness in the face.

Useful to treat when any of the following **physical aspects** are indicated:

- All pain where there is heat, burning, redness or throbbing (e.g. headaches and back pain).
- Colds, coughs and influenza.
- Sore throat.
- Earache.
- Labour pains.
- Cystitis.
- All infections that result in inflammation.
- Teething pain.
- Boils.
- Insomnia.

Modalities

Better: for sitting up.
Worse: for noise and movement.

Treatment tips

An excellent remedy for acute complaints, particularly when accompanied by hot, throbbing sensations. It can be used to lower a temperature.

It is suggested that you add this remedy to your homeopathic first aid kit.

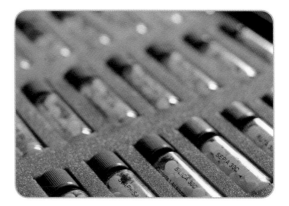

Bryonia

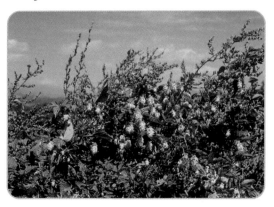

Derived from: wild hops grown in central and southern Europe. The root is used for the remedy. Used by the Romans to treat coughs and wounds.

Useful to treat when any of the following **mental/emotional aspects** are indicated:

- Angry and irritable.
- Needs to be left alone, particularly when unwell.
- Irritability and restlessness.
- Memory is poor.
- Fear of death.

Useful to treat when any of the following **physical aspects** are indicated:

- Headaches, with a bursting or splitting sensation.
- Arthritis and rheumatism.
- Dry eyes and lips.
- Very dry and sore throat.
- Constipation.
- Influenza.
- Very dry, irritating cough.

Modalities

Better: for rest and stillness; cold environment.
Worse: with any kind of movement; cold winds.

Treatment tips

Best used when there is pain on the slightest movement. Most effective when colds are accompanied with a strong thirst and a very dry throat.

Calc. Carb.

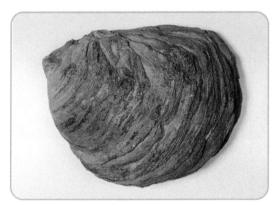

Derived from: calcium carbonate, from the oyster shell.

Useful to treat when any of the following **mental/emotional aspects** are indicated:

- Many types of fears, including of the dark, death, insanity and impending doom.
- In the elderly, fear of a stroke.
- Anxiety, which can cause palpitations.

- Tired, lethargic depression.
- Forgets things easily.
- Tiredness and slowness of thought.
- Obsessed with problems.
- Anxious when criticized.
- Restlessness brought on by fear.
- Hypochondria.
- Jealousy.
- Laziness (particularly with work or exercise).
- Fear of disease.
- Feelings of lowness of spirit.

Useful to treat when any of the following **physical aspects** are indicated:

- Joint and bone pain.
- Fractures, when slow to heal.
- Back pain, with feelings of strain.
- Digestive problems.
- IBS (irritable bowel syndrome).
- Constipation.
- PMS (premenstrual syndrome).
- Nasal congestion, in particular catarrh.
- Polyps.
- Dry and irritating cough.
- Obesity.
- Eating disorders, in particular bulimia.
- Chronic fatigue syndrome.
- TATT (tired all the time).
- Warts.
- Headaches, through study, or when head feels heavy.
- Eye sensitivity to light.
- Loss of hearing.
- Dark rings around the eyes.
- Sour taste in the mouth.
- Bleeding gums.
- Toothache.
- Cramp.
- Tickling cough.
- Stiff neck.
- Weakness in the knees.
- Unhealthy-looking skin.

Modalities

Better: for warm weather.
Worse: in a cold, damp environment or with exertion.

Treatment tips

An excellent remedy when bones are slow to heal.

Calc. Phos.

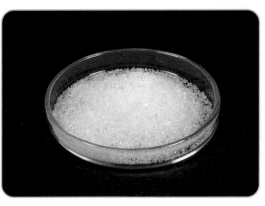

Derived from: the mineral salt calcium phosphate.

Useful to treat when any of the following **mental/emotional aspects** are indicated:

- Unhappiness and discontentment with life, possibly stemming from childhood.
- Prone to irritability.
- Can complain a lot.
- Tendency to become restless.
- Difficulty keeping to routines.
- Constantly need new things to stimulate them.

Useful to treat when any of the following **physical aspects** are indicated:

- Poor memory.
- Illness triggered by relationship break-up.
- All bone and teeth problems, in particular when bones are slow to heal.
- Breaks, fractures and painful joints.
- Slow bone growth with children and teenagers.
- Convalescence, exhaustion and fatigue.
- Digestive disorders.
- Recurrent throat problems.
- Delayed tooth growth in children.

Modalities

Better: for warm, dry, sunny weather.
Worse: in the cold or damp; for stress and worry.

Treatment tips

A good remedy if healing is slow or for any bone and joint complaints.

Cantharis

Derived from: a bright-green beetle known as the Spanish fly. Known for its poisonous and irritant properties since ancient times.

Useful to treat when any of the following **mental/emotional aspects** are indicated:

- Sex addiction.
- Irritability and anger, leading to rage and violence.
- Screaming through anger.

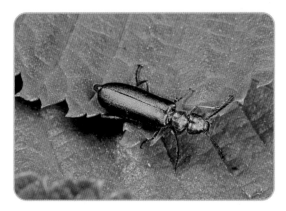

Useful to treat when any of the following **physical aspects** are indicated:

- Severe anxiety.
- All conditions where there is stinging, burning, itching and pain.
- Cystitis and all urinary tract infections, with pain when urinating.
- Burns.
- Diarrhoea with burning sensation.
- Insect stings and bites.
- Burning sore throat.
- Sore, stinging eyes.
- Hot, aching sensation of the stomach.
- Sunburn and inflammation of the skin.

Modalities

Better: for gentle rubbing. **Worse:** for movement and touch.

Carbo Veg.

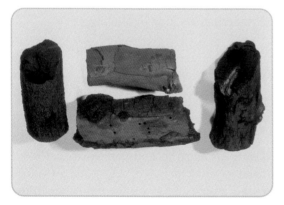

Derived from: vegetable charcoal made from beech, birch or poplar wood. In the past vegetable charcoal was used to absorb gases and help with flatulence.

Useful to treat when any of the following **mental/emotional aspects** are indicated:

Treatment tips

Excellent remedy for treatment of cystitis, especially when the condition worsens without warning.

It is suggested that you add this remedy to your homeopathic first aid kit.

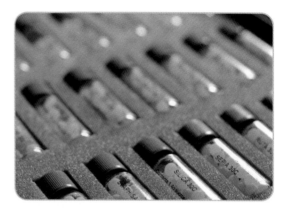

- Loss of memory.
- Fear of strangers.
- Claustrophobia.
- Acute shock.
- Extreme mental exhaustion.
- Feelings of mental and emotional weakness.

Useful to treat when any of the following **physical aspects** are indicated:

- Poor circulation.
- Varicose veins.
- Indigestion.
- Flatulence.

31

- Headaches after too much food.
- Headaches with sickness.
- Coughing.
- Feelings of abdominal bloating (even after eating only small amounts).
- Hoarseness and dryness of the throat.
- Nosebleeds.
- Prolonged illness.

Modalities

Better: for cool, fresh air.
Worse: for fatty foods and in the evening.

Treatment tips

A very good remedy for feeling overtired and run down. Useful after any operation or illness. Good for aiding a slow recovery.

Causticum

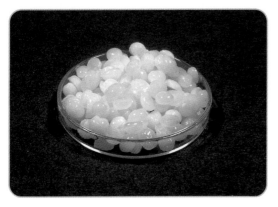

Derived from: a potassium compound commonly called potassium hydrate, prepared from burnt lime, potassium and water.

Useful to treat when any of the following **mental/emotional aspects** are indicated:

- Overcritical of everything.
- Melancholy mood, which may lead to feeling anxious and depressed.
- Children who are excitable and want to get involved in everything.

Useful to treat when any of the following **physical aspects** are indicated:

- Dizziness.

- Heartburn in pregnancy.
- Hoarseness in the throat in the morning.
- Coughs and respiratory conditions.
- Weakness of nerves and muscles, particularly in the bladder.
- Stress incontinence.
- Bed-wetting.
- Leakage of urine when coughing, sneezing, walking or laughing.
- Early periods, with a scanty flow.
- Warts and verrucas.

Modalities

Better: for warmth and damp weather; cold drinks.
Worse: after exercise; on the right side; in the evening.

Treatment tips

Excellent remedy for stress incontinence.

Chamomilla

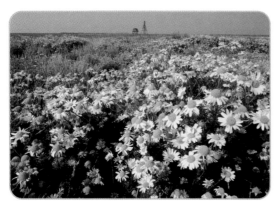

Derived from: the whole, fresh chamomile plant. Used throughout history for its calming, soothing and healing abilities, particularly with skin conditions.

Useful to treat when any of the following **mental/emotional aspects** are indicated:

- Angry when unwell.
- Irritability and whining.
- Impatience.
- Very sensitive and easily upset.
- Spiteful.
- Prone to bad temper and snapping when unwell.

Useful to treat when any of the following **physical aspects** are indicated:

- Earache.
- Toothache.
- Insomnia.
- All skin conditions, including very dry skin, eczema and contact dermatitis.
- Inflamed skin.
- Sleeplessness and colic in children.
- Diarrhoea.
- Coughing, particularly when sleeping.

Modalities

Better: for mild weather.
Worse: for heat and when angry.

Treatment tips

Especially good remedy for the treatment of babies and children. Remember, the Chamomilla child can be oversensitive and always wants to be picked up.

It is suggested that you add this remedy to your homeopathic first aid kit.

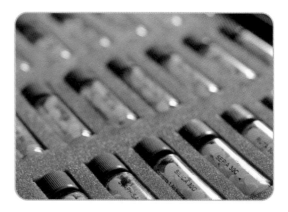

China

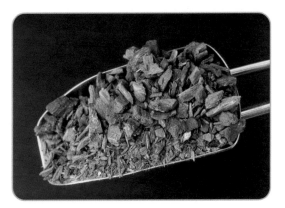

Derived from: Peruvian bark, which contains quinine, one of the first remedies used by Samuel Hahnemann to treat malaria.

Useful to treat when any of the following **mental/emotional aspects** are indicated:

- Feelings of indifference and apathy.
- Nervous exhaustion.
- Feelings of despair.
- Fear of creeping, crawling creatures.
- Angry outbursts.
- Can be deliberately spiteful.
- Can burst into tears suddenly and unexpectedly.
- Depression.
- Eating disorders (anorexia, bulimia).
- Lack of concentration.
- Feelings of being on edge.
- Alcoholism.
- Hypersensitivity.
- Difficulty in self-expression.
- Imaginative.

Useful to treat when any of the following **physical aspects** are indicated:

- Loss of body fluid through heatstroke.
- Diarrhoea.
- Heavy sweating.
- Vomiting.
- Headaches.
- Dizziness.
- Twitches.
- Tiredness and fatigue.
- Nosebleeds.
- Tinnitus.
- Shivering.
- Digestive problems.
- Feelings of coldness.
- Tender scalp.
- Chronic fatigue syndrome.
- Post-viral exhaustion.
- Swollen ankles.
- Fluid retention.
- Gall bladder and gastric complaints.
- Skin that is sensitive to the touch.

Modalities

Better: for warmth and sleep.
Worse: for losing bodily fluids; from cold and draughts.

Treatment tips

A good remedy for feelings of burnout from overwork or emotional traumas that produce feelings of exhaustion and weakness. Also a good convalescent remedy.

Coffea

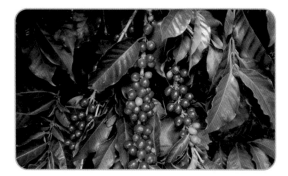

Derived from: caffeine. Used for pain relief, as a stimulant and for digestive disorders. The unroasted coffee bean is used.

Useful to treat when any of the following **mental/emotional aspects** are indicated:

- Hyperactivity and inability to rest the mind.
- Insomnia.
- Overexcitement in children.
- Anxiety and feelings of irritability.
- Sensory overload.
- Feelings of guilt, particularly with children.

Useful to treat when any of the following **physical aspects** are indicated:

- Sensitive reaction to pain.
- Headaches.
- Facial pain and neuralgia.
- Palpitations through anger or stress.

Modalities

Better: for warmth.
Worse: for the open air and strong smells.

Treatment tips

A good remedy for insomnia, particularly when combined with inability to relax or switch off.

Cuprum Met.

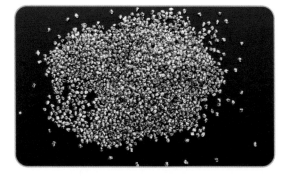

Derived from: the metal copper.

Useful to treat when any of the following **mental/emotional aspects** are indicated:

- Tiredness and exhaustion of the senses.
- Mood changes from a passive to a dominant personality.
- Can sulk when not well.
- Suppression of emotions.
- Self-critical.
- Difficulty expressing true feelings.
- Easily tired, yet driven to continue.
- Fear of strangers.
- Prone to fixed outlook on life.
- Facial twitches through stress.

Useful to treat when any of the following **physical aspects** are indicated:

- All forms of cramp.
- Muscle spasms.
- Constriction, discomfort and pain in the limbs.
- Bad taste in the mouth, in particular a metallic-type taste.
- Dry lips.
- Neuralgia.
- Finger cramps, through writing or typing.
- Prone to nausea and stomach upsets.
- Post-viral fatigue syndrome.

- TATT (tired all the time).
- Respiratory problems, in particular asthma and spasmodic coughs.

Modalities

Better: for cold drinks; perspiring.
Worse: at night and for not expressing emotions.

Treatment tips

The first remedy to use with all forms of cramp, in particular if accompanied by spasmodic episodes and pain.

Drosera

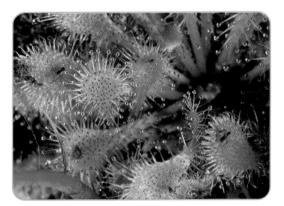

Derived from: the sundew, a tiny plant that traps insects inside its leaves.

Useful to treat when any of the following **mental/emotional aspects** are indicated:

- Feelings of restlessness and anxiety when left alone.
- Fear of ghosts.
- Difficulty concentrating.

Useful to treat when any of the following **physical aspects** are indicated:

- Coughs and colds.
- Coughs that will not stop and are spasmodic.
- A cough that creates a feeling of sickness or vomiting.
- Whooping cough.
- Joint pain and growing pains in the legs of teenagers, if accompanied by symptoms of stiffness.

Modalities

Better: for being outside in the fresh air.
Worse: for lying down.

Treatment tips

An excellent remedy for coughs and colds, in particular for a dry, retching cough.

Gelsemium

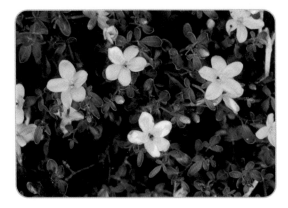

Derived from: the yellow jasmine plant.

Useful to treat when any of the following **mental/emotional aspects** are indicated:

- Fears and phobias when accompanied by shaking and trembling.
- Fear of dentists, doctors, and so on.
- Fear of being left alone.
- Fear and anxiety about forthcoming events, such as meetings.
- Drowsiness and confusion.
- Panic attacks.
- Dislike of insects and things that creep and crawl.
- Difficulty sleeping.

Useful to treat when any of the following **physical aspects** are indicated:

- Influenza.
- Sore throat.
- Tiredness, exhaustion and drowsiness.
- Coughs and colds.
- Shivering.
- Diarrhoea made worse when anxious.
- Migraine and headaches, in particular at the base of the skull or the back of the head.
- Sneezing, with a hot and flushed face.
- Sore, inflamed eyes.
- Weakness and heaviness in the extremities.

Modalities

Better: for rest and stillness; after going to the toilet.
Worse: for cold, damp weather.

Treatment tips

The main influenza remedy. Also excellent for coughs, colds and sore throats, particularly if accompanied by shivering and fever.

It is suggested that you add this remedy to your homeopathic first aid kit.

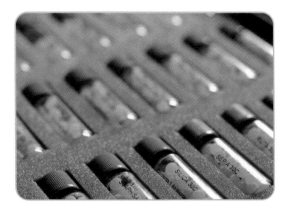

Graphites

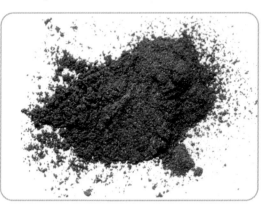

Derived from: the mineral graphite or black lead. Commonly used for pencils.

Useful to treat when any of the following **mental/emotional aspects** are indicated:

- Fidgeting, in particular when nervous and anxious.
- Easily made to feel guilty.
- Depression.
- Indecisiveness.
- Timidness.
- Post-menopausal depression.
- Bulimia.

Useful to treat when any of the following **physical aspects** are indicated:

- Eczema, particularly behind the knees, on the wrists or on the inside and outside of ears.
- Contact dermatitis, particularly on the palms of the hands and between the fingers.
- Very dry skin.
- Psoriasis.
- Dry, cracked and sore skin.

- Cold sores.
- Stomach problems.
- Cramp.
- Constipation.
- Styes.
- Nail problems.
- Chilblains.
- Erratic menstrual cycle.
- Morning headaches.
- Itchiness or skin eruptions of the scalp.

Modalities

Better: for eating.
Worse: for heat.

Treatment tips

Use for the first breakout of skin complaints, in particular eczema and dermatitis. In these cases it should be supported topically with an application of the homeopathic ointment or cream.

It is suggested that you add this remedy to your homeopathic first aid kit.

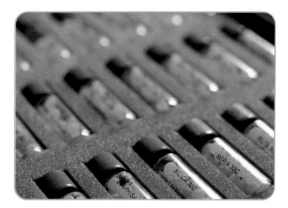

Hamamelis

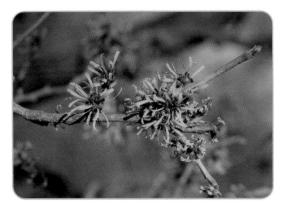

Derived from: the witch hazel plant. The twigs and bark are used.

Useful to treat when any of the following **mental/emotional aspects** are indicated:

- Mild depression, when the person feels better when left alone.
- Irritability and restlessness.
- Irritated by the presence of others.

Useful to treat when any of the following **physical aspects** are indicated:

- Varicose veins.
- Haemorrhoids.
- Useful in the early stages of varicose veins when there is a lack of elasticity in the vein walls.
- Heavy and tired legs.
- Throbbing and itching legs.
- Stinging and aching legs.
- Chilblains.
- Nosebleeds.
- Irritated and bloodshot eyes.
- Bruising around the eyes or a black eye.
- Bruising in general.
- Bleeding, both internal and external (it slows it down).
- Mild skin rashes.
- Insect bites, where accompanied by stinging and aching around the bite.
- Mild burns.
- Acne and oily skin.
- Variocele (varicose veins in the testes).

Modalities

Better: for fresh air.
Worse: for heat and pressure.

Treatment tips

Use at the first sign of varicose veins or haemorrhoids or when these conditions become worse. Can be backed up with a topically applied cream or ointment directly onto the affected sites.

Hepar Sulph.

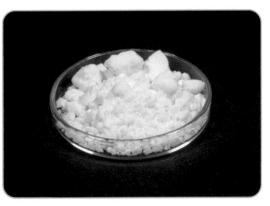

Derived from: calcium sulphide.

Useful to treat when any of the following **mental/emotional aspects** are indicated:

- Irritable over the slightest matter.
- Becomes offended easily.
- Talks quickly when anxious.
- Overreacts when angry.
- Prone to a grumpy nature.
- Can dwell on matters and become resentful.
- Prone to bouts of sadness and depression.

Useful to treat when any of the following **physical aspects** are indicated:

- All skin problems that gather pus and are slow to heal.
- Acne and boils.
- Earache.
- Ear pain with a sore throat.
- Catarrh.
- Coughs that create a hoarse and dry throat.
- Cold sores, particularly around the eyes.
- Mouth ulcers.
- Influenza, with sweating and sneezing.
- Cracked, dry lips.
- Perspiration that causes a bad odour, even when deodorant is used.
- Skin problems that become infected and create a discharge.
- Ulcers on the skin, and bedsores.

Modalities

Better: for warmth and for wrapping up and keeping the head warm.
Worse: for touch and the cold.

Treatment tips

A good remedy to use when things are slow to heal. Good for clearing infections and discharges.

Hypericum

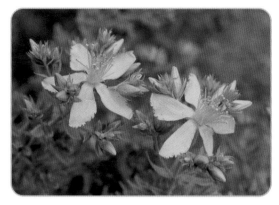

Derived from: the St John's wort herb.

Useful to treat when any of the following **mental/emotional aspects** are indicated:

- Depression, with tiredness and lethargy.
- Depression after surgery or after injury, wounds, and so on.
- Vertigo.
- Shock through injury or emotional trauma.
- Stress and anxiety that causes spasms and feelings of tightness in the body.

Useful to treat when any of the following **physical aspects** are indicated:

- Neuralgia.
- Puncture wounds received from sharp objects (glass, nails, etc.).
- All wounds and injuries, in particular if crushing is involved.
- Concussion.
- Nerve pain or stabbing, shooting pains.
- Injuries to the feet, hands and spine.
- Minor eye injuries.
- Chronic back pain, with a sensation of pain travelling up and down the back.
- Splinters.
- Asthma, when in a damp environment.
- Pain from toothache and dental procedures.
- Diarrhoea.
- Haemorrhoids, with pain and bleeding.

Modalities

Better: for resting the head bent backwards; gentle massage.
Worse: for cold, damp and foggy weather.

Treatment tips

A good remedy to use after an injury or when the skin has been cut and damaged, particularly when there is a risk of infection.

It is suggested that you add this remedy to your homeopathic first aid kit.

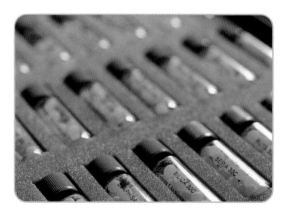

Ignatia

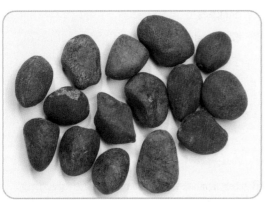

Derived from: St Ignatius bean, a seedpod from the Ignatia Amara tree.

Useful to treat when any of the following **mental/emotional aspects** are indicated:

- Highly emotional states.
- Shock.
- Anger.
- Loss of a loved one and grief.
- Inability to express emotions.
- Reactions of hysteria.
- Insomnia.
- Quick, sudden tearfulness.
- Self-blame and pity.
- Worry.
- Divorce and broken relationships.
- Sudden, unexpected mood changes.
- Overburdened with work, leading to exhaustion.
- Obsessive compulsive behaviour.
- Hypochondria.
- Jealousy.
- Fixed ideas.

Useful to treat when any of the following **physical aspects** are indicated:

- Headaches caused by emotional stress and tension.
- Coughs and sore throats.
- Difficulty swallowing.
- Twitching of the face, when caused by anxiety.
- Stomach and digestive problems, in particular after shock or grief, when accompanied with a 'sinking sensation'.
- Diarrhoea.
- Disruptive sleep patterns, particularly if grieving.

Modalities

Better: for warmth and the sun; change of position.
Worse: for emotional upset; in the morning.

Treatment tips

One of the best remedies for emotional problems. It is good for mood swings, bereavement and the physical ailments they can bring. Also particularly good if the ailments are very changeable.

Ipecac.

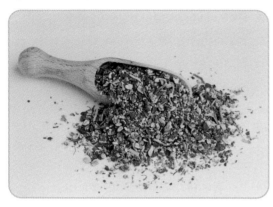

Derived from: the small shrub called Cephaelis ipecacuanha, which grows in rainforests. The dried root is used to make the remedy.

Useful to treat when any of the following **mental/emotional aspects** are indicated:

- Anxiety.
- Worry.
- Fear of death.
- Sulkiness.
- Glumness.

Useful to treat when any of the following **physical aspects** are indicated:

- Dry, spasmodic cough.
- Respiratory conditions.
- Nausea from headaches.
- Sickness.
- Stomach upsets.
- Fainting.
- Asthma.
- Travel sickness and motion sickness.

Modalities

Better: for fresh air; being in the open; rest.
Worse: for motion; movement; warmth and heat; stress.

Treatment tips

Excellent for all forms of travel sickness (boat, car, plane, etc.). Especially good with the individual who is full of anxiety.

It is suggested that you add this remedy to your homeopathic first aid kit.

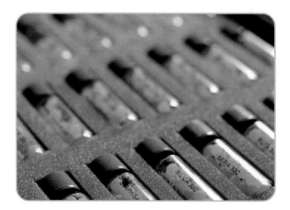

Kali Phos.

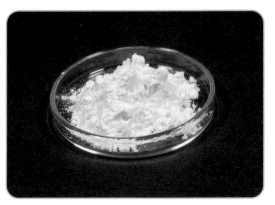

Derived from: potassium phosphate.

Useful to treat when any of the following **mental/emotional aspects** are indicated:

- Complete exhaustion.
- Oversensitive reactions and nervousness when stressed.
- Overwhelmed by study or recall of information.
- Shyness and withdrawal when anxious.
- Prone to frustration due to lack of self-assertiveness.
- Nervous when meeting people.
- Can become depressed.
- Nightmares.
- Lack of concentration and weak memory.
- Fear of a nervous breakdown.
- Post-viral depression.

Useful to treat when any of the following **physical aspects** are indicated:

- Weakness of limbs.
- Neck and upper back pain.
- Headaches caused by tension.
- Dizziness when standing, from sitting or kneeling.
- Chronic fatigue syndrome.
- Discharges from colds and catarrh.
- Productive coughs.
- Diarrhoea.
- Cystitis.

Modalities

Better: for heat and movement.
Worse: for worry; meeting deadlines.

Treatment tips

Known as the great nerve soother, it is excellent with all forms of exhaustion, particularly if brought about by stress.

Lachesis

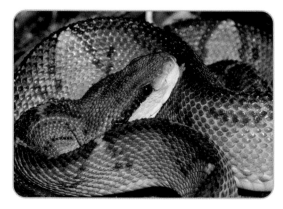

Derived from: the venom of the bushmaster snake. The bushmaster is a very aggressive snake, with a deadly venom.

Useful to treat when any of the following **mental/emotional aspects** are indicated:

- Hypersensitivity.
- Very talkative.
- Rambling, self-absorbed nature.
- Restlessness.
- Fixed ideas and opinions, in particular about religion and beliefs.
- Fear of personal attack or burglary.
- Suspicious of new people.
- Jealous and suspicious of loved ones.
- Suppression of anger.
- Post-menopausal depression.
- Nightmares.
- Irritability.
- Anger after the break-up of relationships.
- Addictions, including alcohol, tobacco and drugs.
- Premenstrual syndrome.
- Panic attacks.
- No desire to mix with the world.

Useful to treat when any of the following **physical aspects** are indicated:

- Headaches, particularly when waking.
- Nosebleeds.
- Puffy, bloated or swollen face.
- Stomach ache when craving stimulants.
- Constrictive, sore throat.
- Asthma.
- Angina pain.
- Palpitations and tightness or constriction of the chest.
- Menopause.
- Hot flushes.
- Feeling bloated.
- Varicose veins.
- Haemorrhoids.
- Variocele.
- Phlebitis and thrombosis.

Modalities

Better: in the open air; cool drinks.
Worse: when trying to sleep; from touch; tight clothing.

Treatment tips

Excellent for all circulatory problems. Also good for extreme stress when accompanied by pains and tightness in the chest.

Ledum

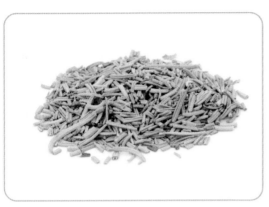

Derived from: dried wild rosemary plant.

Useful to treat when any of the following **mental/emotional aspects** are indicated:

- Feelings of hotness and swelling, triggered by stress.
- Sleep disturbance, with night sweats.
- Impatience.
- Timidity.

Useful to treat when any of the following **physical aspects** are indicated:

- Wounds.
- Stings with bruising and puffiness.
- Grazes and cuts.
- Bites.
- Infection through cuts, bites or stings.
- Injury to the eyes.

- Arthritic and rheumatic pain when affecting the lower limbs (ankles, knees and lower legs).
- Hot, burning sensations in the limbs.
- Gout.

Modalities

Better: for cold compresses.
Worse: at night and with heat.

Treatment tips

This is an ideal 'puncture' remedy. It can prevent any infection caused by bites, stings, cuts, and so on.

It is suggested that you add this remedy to your homeopathic first aid kit.

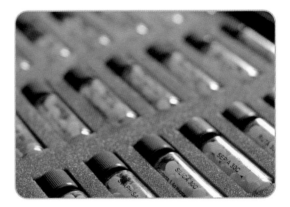

Lycopodium

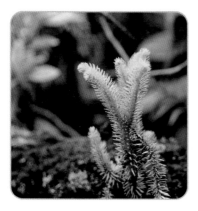

Derived from: the pollen dust from an evergreen herb.

Useful to treat when any of the following **mental/emotional aspects** are indicated:

- Lack of self-confidence.
- Sexual fears.
- Anxiety and fear of interviews and speeches.
- Sensitive personality.
- Forgetfulness.
- Irritated by small things.
- Dislikes contradictions.
- Feelings of stress when meeting strangers.
- Fear of ghosts, death and the dark.
- Does not like being alone.
- Suppresses fears.
- Agoraphobia.
- Nervous breakdown.
- Bulimia.

Useful to treat when any of the following **physical aspects** are indicated:

- Digestive disorders, such as indigestion, IBS, feelings of nausea, ulcers and hunger pains.
- Feels bloated after small amounts of food.
- Flatulence.
- Constipation.
- Impotence.
- Sore throats.
- Dry cough.
- Extreme tiredness, followed by colds or influenza.
- Chronic fatigue syndrome.
- Bladder and kidney problems (including kidney stones).
- Prostate problems.
- Hair loss.
- Restless legs at night.
- Cold hands and feet.
- Headaches over the eyes.
- Shoulder pain.
- Varicose veins.
- Eczema, when chronic.

Modalities

Better: for small meals and movement.
Worse: for heat and stuffy environment.

Treatment tips

The first remedy to use for digestive disorders, including IBS.

Merc. Sol.

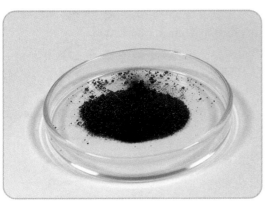

Derived from: the black oxide of mercury.

Useful to treat when any of the following **mental/emotional aspects** are indicated:

- Sluggishness of thought.
- Distrustful of others.
- Fear of burglary and abuse.
- Poor memory and difficulty in recall.
- Mental and emotional weakness and fatigue.
- Restlessness and anxiousness.
- Deep insecurity.
- Suspicious of motives.
- Sensitive to criticism.
- Quick, sudden and aggressive temper.
- Weak will-power.
- Tendency to be arrogant.
- Emotionally repressed.

Useful to treat when any of the following **physical aspects** are indicated:

- Stammering.
- Dribbling from the mouth when snoozing.
- Tiredness in the limbs and feelings of weakness through the whole body.
- Chronic fatigue syndrome.
- Body odour.
- Bad taste in the mouth, in particular a metallic taste.
- Cutting, burning pain.
- Gum and mouth problems.
- Sore throats.
- Mouth ulcers.
- Bedsores.
- Oral thrush.
- Spasmodic coughs.
- Joint pain.
- Conjunctivitis with discharge.
- Catarrh.
- Scalp problems, eruptions and crustiness of the scalp.
- Cold sores.

Modalities

Better: for rest.
Worse: at night; for heat.

Treatment tips

An excellent remedy for oral problems, especially mouth ulcers and gum problems.

Nat. Mur.

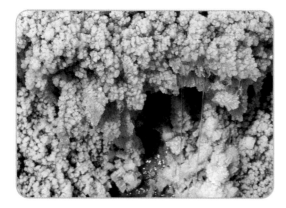

Derived from: the mineral rock salt or sodium chloride.

Useful to treat when any of the following **mental/emotional aspects** are indicated:

- Anxiety and depression caused by suppressed grief.
- Repressed fear.
- Agoraphobia.
- Fear of thunderstorms.
- Hypochondria.
- Agitation.
- Guilt.
- Anorexia.
- Shock.
- Low self-worth.
- Premenstrual syndrome.
- Quick changing of emotions, without warning.
- Resentment.
- Tendency to sulk or keep feelings locked away.

Useful to treat when any of the following **physical aspects** are indicated:

- Sunstroke.
- Migraine.
- Eye strain.
- Cold sores.
- Cracked and dry lips.
- Mouth ulcers.
- Inflamed gums.
- Boils and warts.
- Anaemia.
- Constipation.
- Backache.
- Irregular periods.
- Hair loss.
- Oily skin and hair.
- Coughs and colds.
- Palpitations.

Modalities

Better: for cool, fresh air.
Worse: for heat and strong sunlight; on waking.

Treatment tips

A good remedy for people who brood on the past. Very good for loss, grief and separation.

Nux Vomica

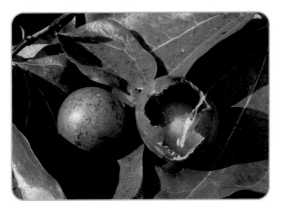

Derived from: strychnine, extracted from the seeds of the Strychnos nux vomica tree.

Useful to treat when any of the following **mental/emotional aspects** are indicated:

- Tendency to overindulge.
- Cravings for stimulants, such as alcohol, tobacco or rich food.
- Addictive personality types.
- Finicky and fussy.
- Fear of failure.
- Argumentative and quarrelsome.
- Critical.
- Fear and hate of small insects, such as spiders and beetles.
- Dread of death.
- Depression.
- Insomnia.
- Hyperactivity.
- Frustration.

Useful to treat when any of the following **physical aspects** are indicated:

- Headaches and migraines.
- All stomach problems, in particular indigestion and heartburn.
- Gastric problems caused by too much food and drink.
- Food poisoning.
- Vomiting.
- Constipation.
- Diarrhoea.
- Lower back pain.
- Hernias.
- Hiccups.
- Hay fever.
- Coughs, colds and influenza.
- Stomach cramps.
- Blocked nose.
- Heavy, aching muscles.
- Body feels weak and fragile.
- Heavy periods.
- Morning sickness and cramp in pregnancy.

Modalities

Better: for sleep.
Worse: in the morning.

Treatment tips

Known as the hangover remedy. Excellent for any form of excess caused by food and drink. Also good for aiding digestion and promoting the appetite.

It is suggested that you add this remedy to your homeopathic first aid kit.

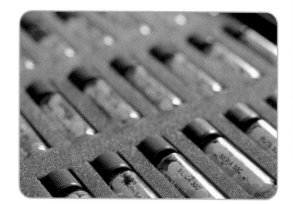

Petroleum

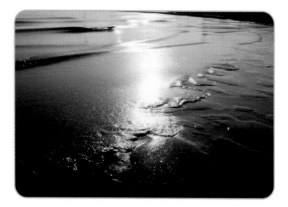

Derived from: crude rock oil that lies beneath the earth's surface. The purified crude oil is used to make the remedy.

Useful to treat when any of the following **mental/emotional aspects** are indicated:

- Excitable.
- Irritable and quarrelsome.

Useful to treat when any of the following **physical aspects** are indicated:

- Very dry skin conditions.
- Cracks in the skin.
- Rough texture to the skin.
- Tips of the fingers and hands are dry and irritated.
- Eczema and dermatitis.
- Skin worsening in the winter months.

Modalities

Better: for dry, warm weather and air.
Worse: for cold weather; travel.

Treatment tips

Remedy of choice when the skin is extremely dry and cracked.

Phosphorus

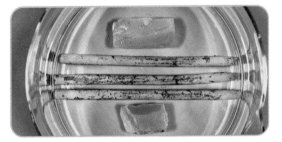

Derived from: a mineral found in phosphates and living matter. Contained in bones, teeth and bodily fluids.

Useful to treat when any of the following **mental/emotional aspects** are indicated:

- Hypersensitivity.
- Imaginative.
- Angers easily.
- Fearful, particularly of darkness and death.
- Keeps fear suppressed.
- Fixed ideas.
- Fatigue.
- Craves reassurance.
- Worried unnecessarily about health.
- Nightmares and insomnia.
- Facial twitches.
- Shock.
- Low spirit.
- Clairvoyant episodes.
- Panic attacks.
- Prefers company and fears loneliness.

Useful to treat when any of the following **physical aspects** are indicated:

- Unproductive, hard, dry cough, with a tight, heavy chest.
- Low resistance to infections such as colds and influenza.
- Always feels the cold.
- Asthma.
- Bruising.
- Headaches.
- Vertigo.
- Styes.
- Exhaustion and fatigue.
- Nosebleeds.
- Gums that bleed.
- Heavy periods.
- Food poisoning.
- Heartburn.
- Pneumonia.
- Bronchitis.
- Back pain expressed through a burning, hot sensation.
- Sore throat, with hoarseness.
- Dandruff.
- Weakness in the extremities.

Modalities

Better: for warm, fresh air; for touch and rubbing.
Worse: for overexertion; at night.

Treatment tips

When ailments and emotional states are brought about by fear and anxiety, this is an ideal remedy as it treats the nervous system very effectively.

Pulsatilla

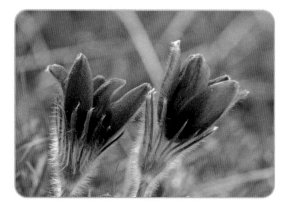

Derived from: the Pulsatilla plant, native to Scandinavia, Germany and Russia. The fresh plant in flower is used.

Useful to treat when any of the following **mental/emotional aspects** are indicated:

- Tendency to weep and burst into tears without warning.
- Mild, gentle temperament.
- Prone to quietness.
- Suppression of fear.
- Depression.
- Obsessive compulsive behaviour.
- Fear of the opposite sex.
- Fear of the dark and ghosts.
- Grief with lots of tears.
- Bulimia.

Useful to treat when any of the following **physical aspects** are indicated:

- Coughs and colds.
- Runny nose.
- Catarrh.
- Conjunctivitis.
- Digestive problems.
- All menstrual problems and menopausal problems, particularly if accompanied by depression.
- Lower back pain.
- Headaches.
- Varicose veins.
- Arthritis.
- Styes.
- Incontinence.
- IBS.
- Skin problems.

Modalities

Better: for crying; for cool, fresh air.
Worse: for heat.

Treatment tips

This remedy works well on the mental state of the individual.

Rhus Tox.

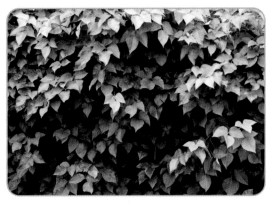

Derived from: the fresh leaves of the poison ivy plant.

Useful to treat when any of the following **mental/emotional aspects** are indicated:

- Irritability.
- Depression.
- Suicidal thoughts.
- Lack of joy in life.
- Anxiousness.
- Fear of being poisoned.
- Anxiety at night.

Useful to treat when any of the following **physical aspects** are indicated:

- Skin problems, eczema and dermatitis.
- Skin-blistering problems.
- Burning, itching, swollen skin.
- Cold sores and all other herpes-related conditions.
- Nappy rash.
- Sciatica.
- Chickenpox.
- Shingles.
- Influenza and other viral infections.
- Dizziness.
- Sore, stinging eyes.
- Heavy, prolonged periods.
- Muscular aches and pains.
- Stiffness.
- Joint pain.
- Back pain.
- Arthritis and rheumatism.
- Sprains and strains.
- Jaw pain.
- Frozen shoulder.
- Neuralgia.
- Post-operative recovery where there is pain and stiffness.
- RSI (repetitive strain injury).

Modalities

Better: for movement; for a warm, dry atmosphere.
Worse: for rest and stillness; for cold, damp weather.

Treatment tips

Excellent remedy for muscular aches and pains. Particularly good if condition is improved through movement. Eczema and other skin problems often respond to this remedy where others fail.

It is suggested that you add this remedy to your homeopathic first aid kit.

Ruta Grav.

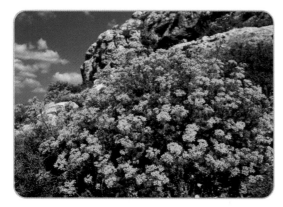

Derived from: the Ruta graveolens herb. The juice from the whole plant, before it flowers, is used.

Useful to treat when any of the following **mental/emotional aspects** are indicated:

- Low personal satisfaction.
- Depression.
- Critical of others and self.
- Anxiousness.

Useful to treat when any of the following **physical aspects** are indicated:

- Aches and pains in bones and muscles.
- Deep, aching pain.
- Arthritis and rheumatism.
- RSI (repetitive strain injury).
- Injuries to ligaments, tendons and cartilage.
- Sciatic pain.

- Chest and rib pain caused from the strain of coughing.
- Eye strain and exhaustion from overwork.
- Headaches, in particular from reading.
- Constipation.

Modalities

Better: for movement.
Worse: for cold damp weather; for lying down.

Treatment tips

This remedy acts upon the periosteum (the lining of the bone) and cartilage, so is excellent for injuries to gliding joints such as the ankle and wrist. This remedy is also the first choice for RSI (repetitive strain injury), which is an inflammation of the tendon sheaths of the arm and wrist.

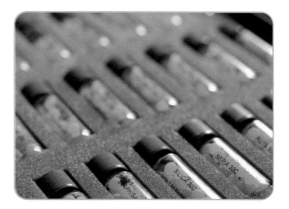

Sepia

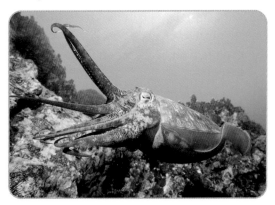

Derived from: the ink from the cuttlefish (related to the octopus and squid).

Useful to treat when any of the following **mental/emotional aspects** are indicated:

- Menopausal depression.
- Exhaustion and slowness of thought.
- Feelings of weakness.
- Tendency to cry easily.
- Stress and anxiety.
- Feelings of being unable to cope.
- Fear of sickness and disease.
- Fixed ideas.
- Irritability.
- Grief.
- Separation and break-up of relationships.

Useful to treat when any of the following **physical aspects** are indicated:

- Chronic fatigue syndrome.
- Menopausal problems – hot flushes and night sweats.
- Headaches and migraines.
- Constipation.
- Haemorrhoids and varicose veins.
- Ovarian, uterine and vaginal complaints.
- Heavy periods.
- Thrush.
- Prolapse of the uterus.
- Backache with weakness.
- Flatulence and abdominal tenderness.
- Hair loss.
- Tiredness.
- Dizziness.
- Sweaty feet.

Modalities

Better: for sleep; for warmth; for gentle exercise.

Worse: in the morning; for sedentary lifestyle.

Treatment tips

An excellent 'women's' remedy as it helps greatly with the menopause. Also good for exhaustion and TATT complaints.

Silicea

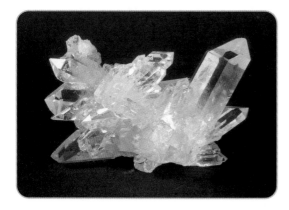

Derived from: the main part of most rocks and plant stems (it helps to keep them strong and upright). Also found in teeth, hair and bones. Quartz or flint are the main derivatives of this remedy, although it can be prepared chemically.

Useful to treat when any of the following **mental/emotional aspects** are indicated:

- Low self-confidence.
- Fear of failure.
- People who lack assertiveness and can be timid.
- Anxiety stemming from important events or interviews.
- Exhaustion after periods of concentration.
- Performance fear.
- Obsessive about detail.
- Stubbornness.
- Anorexia.
- Fear of commitment.

Useful to treat when any of the following **physical aspects** are indicated:

- Feelings of coldness.
- Slowness of healing.
- Recurrent coughs, colds and respiratory infections.
- Sore, throbbing throat.
- Sweaty feet and head.
- Boils.
- Headaches, especially if triggered by a cold atmosphere.
- Chest infections, especially if a family history of tuberculosis.
- Painful joints and bones.
- Constipation.
- Under-nourishment.
- Weak immune system.
- Unhealthy skin, including acne.
- Bones and fractures that are slow to heal.
- Splinters.
- Catarrh.
- Weak nervous system.
- Ear infections.
- Slow bone growth in babies and children.
- Light-sensitivity of the eyes.
- Loss of smell.
- Cracking at the corners of the mouth.
- Sensitive gums.
- Swelling of glands.

Modalities

Better: for keeping warm.
Worse: for cold damp weather and for draughts.

Treatment tips

A good remedy to use if an individual has low resistance to disease and is slow to recover from illness.

Staphisagria

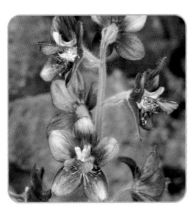

Derived from: the seed of the plant Delphinium staphysagria, commonly known as Staveacre.

Useful to treat when any of the following **mental/emotional aspects** are indicated:

- Suppression of emotions, in particular anger.
- Bursts of temper.
- Fixation about an illness, symptom or emotional problem.
- Likes to be alone.
- Sensitive to criticism and easily offended.
- Resentment and jealousy.
- Hypersensitivity.
- Sex addiction.
- Workaholic.
- Overindulgence of alcohol, tobacco or food.

Useful to treat when any of the following **physical aspects** are indicated:

- Post-operative trauma, healing of wounds after operations.
- Healing after cuts and incisions.
- Enlargement of prostate gland.
- Skin problems.
- Headaches, in particular after arguments.
- Flatulence with a strong smell.
- Teething problems.
- Neuralgia.
- Styes.
- Inflammation of the eyes.

Modalities

Better: for warmth.
Worse: for suppressing emotions; from touch.

Treatment tips

An excellent remedy for treating suppressed emotions and anger, and any diseases that stem from this.

Stramonium

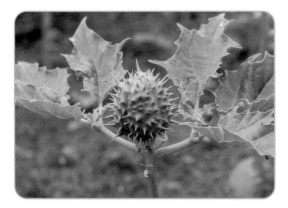

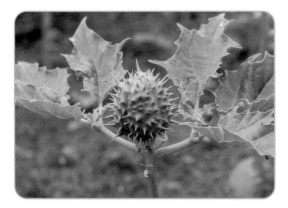

Derived from: the juice of the thorn apple plant.

Useful to treat when any of the following **mental/emotional aspects** are indicated:

- All states of fear, in particular fear of water, darkness, animals and violence.
- Nightmares (especially in children).
- Stammering due to nervousness.
- Talkative.
- Mood swings and quick changes of temper.
- Dislike of own company.
- Jealousy.
- Anger.
- Unable to settle into a new environment (e.g. new home or new job).
- Expressionless.

Useful to treat when any of the following **physical aspects** are indicated:

- Muscular spasms.
- Cramps.
- Convulsions.
- Restless legs accompanied by twitching and jerking.
- Sore throat with a great thirst.
- Hay fever.
- Conditions that are stress-related.

Modalities

Better: for light rooms; for company.
Worse: for darkness; loneliness.

Treatment tips

An excellent remedy for anxious states.

Sulphur

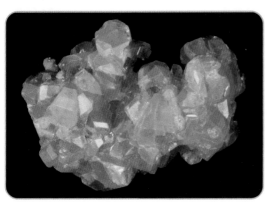

Derived from: the mineral sulphur.

Useful to treat when any of the following **mental/emotional aspects** are indicated:

- Forgetfulness.
- Inability to think clearly.
- Lack of regard for others.
- Lazy.
- Irritable.
- Self-centred and selfish.
- Argumentative.
- Aggressive tendencies.
- Claustrophobia.
- Vertigo.
- Fear of oppression.
- Bulimia.
- Insomnia.
- Post-menopausal depression.
- Alcoholism.
- Smoking addiction.
- Lack of will-power.
- Nightmares.

Useful to treat when any of the following **physical aspects** are indicated:

- Burning, itching skin.
- Eczema, dermatitis or psoriasis.
- Thrush.
- Nappy rash.
- Catarrh.
- Hot, sweaty, burning feet.
- Constipation.
- Diarrhoea.
- Indigestion.
- Loss of appetite.
- Haemorrhoids.
- Lower back pain.
- Gout.
- Digestive disorders.
- Headaches.
- Conjunctivitis.
- Red, sore and itchy eyes.
- Offensive body odour.
- Menopausal problems, such as hot flushes and dizziness.
- Hair loss.
- Dry, itchy scalp.
- Dry lips.
- Sore throat.
- Stiff knees and ankles.

Modalities

Better: for fresh, warm air.
Worse: for washing; for sitting and standing.

Treatment tips

All skin problems, particularly if red and itchy (such as eczema), respond well to this remedy. Also a good general remedy for detoxification.

It is suggested that you add this remedy to your homeopathic first aid kit.

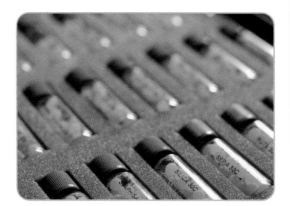

Symphytum

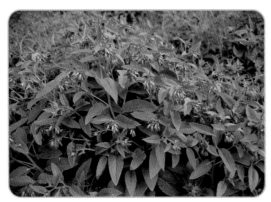

Derived from: the plant comfrey (Symphytum officinale).

Useful to treat when any of the following **mental/emotional aspects** are indicated:

- ✎ None.

Useful to treat when any of the following **physical aspects** are indicated:

- ✎ All fractures.
- ✎ Broken bones, where the bones are slow or difficult to knit.
- ✎ Injuries to the eye or eye socket after a blow to the area.

Modalities

Better: for warmth and rest; stillness.
Worse: for touch and movement; pressure.

Treatment tips

This is known as the bone-knit remedy and is excellent in promoting healing to all bone injuries, particularly fractures. Always make sure the break has been set before introducing this remedy.

Thuja

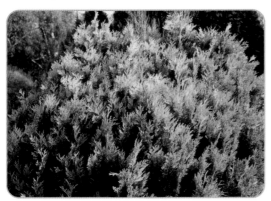

Derived from: the leaves and twigs of the evergreen conifer tree, commonly known as the Arbor vitae or white cedar tree.

Useful to treat when any of the following **mental/emotional aspects** are indicated:

- Anorexia.
- Distorted ideas of body image.
- Fear of strangers.
- Facial twitches.
- Fixed ideas.
- Anxiety.
- Cries and weeps easily.
- Dyslexia.
- Paranoia.
- Poor, interrupted sleep.
- Lack of self-esteem.

- Secretive.
- Manipulative, but weak of character.

Useful to treat when any of the following **physical aspects** are indicated:

- Warts.
- Verrucas.
- Skin complaints.
- Very oily skin.
- Acne.
- Perspiration, with odour.
- Headaches.
- Polyps of the nose.
- Styes.
- Nail problems.
- Haemorrhoids.
- Loss of appetite.
- Constantly cold.

Modalities

Better: for movement.
Worse: for cold, damp environment; at night.

Treatment tips

Always the first remedy of choice for warts and verrucas. Can be applied topically to back up the oral treatment.

Urtica

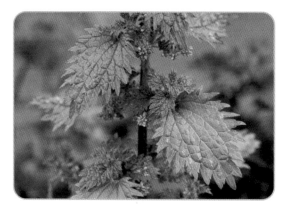

Derived from: the stinging nettle plant, Urtica urens. The whole plant is used in the remedy.

Useful to treat when any of the following **mental/emotional aspects** are indicated:

- When symptoms return at the same time every year, possibly linked with recurring events, such as family reunions, birthdays, anniversaries, yearly appraisals at work.

Useful to treat when any of the following **physical aspects** are indicated:

- Vertigo.
- Gout.
- Individuals who are prone to uric acid build-ups.
- Neuralgia and after nerve inflammation.
- Blotchy, itchy skin.

- When skin is blistered, hot and burning.
- For skin conditions, especially when due to an allergic reaction (e.g. from eating shellfish, insect bites and stings).
- For rashes, hives and eczema, with much itching.
- Also useful for cystitis.

Modalities

Better: for lying down; rubbing irritated area.
Worse: at night; in a cold, damp environment; eating shellfish.

Treatment tips

Good remedy for all stinging, burning, itchy skin complaints. Dose with the remedy as soon as the symptoms occur. Excellent to apply in cream form to calm and soothe a localized area.

It is suggested that you add this remedy to your homeopathic first aid kit.

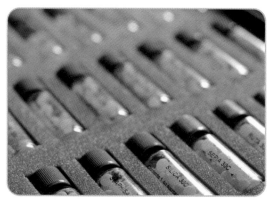

Zinc. Met.

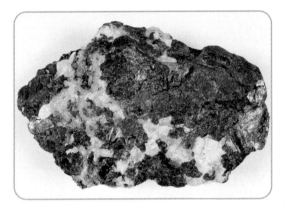

Derived from: zinc sulphide.

Useful to treat when any of the following **mental/emotional aspects** are indicated:

- Weakness and exhaustion.
- Restlessness.
- Always fidgeting.
- Brain fatigue.
- Weak, poor memory.
- Head feels heavy.
- Depression.
- Bulimia.
- Alcoholism.

- Irritability.
- Jumpiness.

Useful to treat when any of the following **physical aspects** are indicated:

- Exhaustion.
- Restless legs.
- Tiredness through lack of sleep.
- Chilblains.
- Cramp.
- Varicose veins.
- Chronic fatigue syndrome.
- Chronic fatigue after viruses.
- Sensitivity to noise.
- Anaemia.

Modalities

Better: for bowel movement; emotional reassurance.
Worse: after food.

Treatment tips

A good remedy for lack of vitality. Also good for feelings of constant coldness or chilliness.

FAQs: Homeopathic remedies

Where can I purchase homeopathic remedies?

My first choice would be a homeopathic pharmacy or known homeopathic supplier. Obtaining a remedy from these sources guarantees the quality, as often the remedies are freshly made up for your order. These suppliers also offer a wider choice of hard or soft tablets, powders, and so on. Health food stores and chemists will also stock a limited range of remedies. You may also see them in supermarkets. If you are under the care of a homeopath, they may dispense the remedies themselves. (See page 155, Where to go from here.)

How should the homeopathic remedies be kept?

Make sure you store them in a cold, dry place, away from direct sunlight. A dark cupboard, away from strong-smelling things, is ideal. Always ensure the top is well screwed on and keep them in their original container. Follow these steps and the remedies will be kept at their optimum strength for the longest period of time.

Can I make my own remedies from my garden, using plants?

The homeopathic remedies are made using a specialized process. It is always advisable to obtain the homeopathic remedies from one of the major suppliers or health food stores. It is also important to buy a well-known and trusted brand. The plants in your garden are more suited to make herbal infusions, teas and massage oils.

Is it possible to put a small kit of remedies together to cover the most common conditions, so that I can take it to work or when travelling?

Yes. For a basic kit, first think which remedies have worked well for you in the past and include them in your kit – remember to select some remedies that have matched your constitution. Then add to this some of the more regularly used remedies, such as Aconite, Belladonna, Hypericum, Nux Vomica, Rhus Tox., Arnica and Cantharis. These remedies would cover general conditions, such as sleeplessness, fear, heatstroke, high temperature, swelling, infection, cuts, wounds, stings and bites. (See Chapter 9: Travel and first aid kit, for more detail.)

homeopathic dos and don'ts

Following these simple dos and don'ts will help you to get the most out of your chosen remedy, as many of the bottles will not have detailed instructions on the label.

Dos

- Try to leave your mouth free from food and liquid 20–30 minutes each side of taking the remedy. This includes cigarettes and brushing your teeth!
- Remember to carry the remedy with you in case you need an extra dose.
- Try to use a homeopathic toothpaste, such as Calendula, as this will be free from substances that may act as an antidote to the remedy.

- Tap the tablet into the lid of the bottle or vial, and then tip it into your mouth, to avoid hand contact.
- Store in a dark, cool place or a remedy box.
- Check the expiry date if you have had the remedy for some time.
- Keep out of reach of children and pets.

Don'ts

- Do not swallow the tablet. You should suck it until it has gone.
- Do not drink coffee while on a course of a remedy, as this may counteract its effectiveness.

- Do not consume mints, peppermints or menthol cough sweets, as this may counteract the effectiveness of the remedy.
- Do not use essential oils, such as camphor, eucalyptus, menthol,

peppermint or rosemary, as this may counteract the effectiveness of the remedy.

- Do not touch the remedy. Always tap the tablets into the lid, as the sweat from your fingertips or palm may absorb the remedy rather than your mouth.

- Do not store remedies near strong-smelling perfume, essential oils, and so on.

- Do not spray perfume 30 minutes either side of taking the remedy.

FAQs: Dos and don'ts

Can I use other forms of complementary therapy alongside my homeopathic treatment?

Yes and no! Massage works well alongside homeopathy, but with a base oil only (i.e. one containing no essential oils). Reflexology is a great choice alongside homeopathy, particularly when the client needs a touch therapy for pain relief, relaxation, stress-related conditions and to help with joint flexibility, and so on. Indian head massage works well alongside both homeopathy and reflexology, as does osteopathy and chiropractic. Acupuncture is also a good complement to a homeopathic treatment. A good general rule of thumb is that all touch therapies can be used alongside homeopathy, as long as essential oils are avoided. I would not recommend using herbal medicine, as this would act as an antidote to the effect of the homeopathic remedies, as would Chinese herbal medicine. Any massage involving essential oils (usually aromatherapy massage) should be avoided, as the strong oils can act as an antidote to the homeopathic remedies. It may be that some oils would work alongside homeopathy, but this would have to be in small quantities and with a full

understanding of the current homeopathic remedy you were taking. It is also important for the homeopath to know which other therapies are being used, so that this can be taken into account in assessing the effectiveness of the overall treatment.

Can I use homeopathy alongside my medical treatment if I am using allopathic medicines, such as anti-inflammatories, insulin or thyroxin?

Absolutely. The homeopathic remedy will not interfere with the effectiveness of the allopathic medication, and can often contribute towards a good therapeutic effect by helping to relieve side effects or other related conditions. For example, a woman who has being taking thyroxin for several years for an underactive thyroid gland may feel less tired, but may still feel low in spirit or mildly depressed from time to time. She may also continue to experience headaches. These symptoms can be treated with a homeopathic remedy alongside her use of thyroxin. In such cases it is important that the patient should seek approval from their doctor or consultant before taking homeopathic remedies.

taking the remedies and prescribing doses

Taking the remedies

- Homeopathic tablets should **not be handled**, because sweat from the fingertips will absorb the potency of the remedy and make it less effective. Tip tablets into the lid of the container and then drop into the mouth. If in powder form, make the wrapping that surrounds the powder into a funnel and tap the powder into the mouth.

- Only one or two tablets should be taken per dose.

- Tablets must be sucked and **not swallowed whole**.

- Tablets are not to be taken within 20–30 minutes of drinking tea or coffee, cold drinks, food, smoking or brushing the teeth.

Doses

The potencies recommended for use with this book are 6c, 30c and 200c.

- **30c** is sufficient for most conditions covered and may also work on a light constitutional level.

- **200c** is higher and will have more effect when treating emotional conditions or when following the 30c. It has a deeper effect at the constitutional level.

- If taking the constitutional remedy, a good starting point is to take one to two tablets up to three times a day at the start of the symptoms or disturbance, or to boost the constitution when feeling weak, tired or run down. Take this dose for up to three days. If improvement begins, stop taking the remedy or cut the dose down to one a day for a few days for

69

further improvement, if you feel it is needed. **Only repeat the dose pattern if the symptoms reappear.**

🔖 A lower dose of **6c** may be taken for a little longer when treating common conditions, as may the 30c at one or two tablets a day.

🔖 A **200c** dose may be taken for deeper emotional problems and when focusing more on the constitution. One to three doses can be prescribed. If prescribing three, they are usually given close together (night, morning, night). Sometimes the dose is repeated after one month. The dosing regime may vary, depending on the individual's circumstances and reactions to treatment.

Remember, the power is in the **minimum** dose. Many people respond well after just one or two doses, and this may be all that is required. **Always stop when improvement has occurred.** In a sudden, acute condition, like a headache, stomach upset, insect bite or sting, administer one dose of 6c or 30c every hour for up to four doses, then monitor for an improvement within several hours. A deeper complaint, like a cold with a

very sore throat, may take up 36 hours or more before real improvement is seen, so the dosage may be reduced after the first four doses to two or three times a day. Often with a bowel condition, like chronic constipation, it may be two to four days before an improvement is seen. If the problem is mild, one tablet taken twice a day can be prescribed until improvement is felt.

Key points

🔖 The **golden rule** of homeopathy is: **only repeat the remedy if the symptoms return**.

🔖 Try not to take the remedy for more than three or four days; if it has not helped within this time then it is usually an indication that another remedy needs to be selected.

🔖 **Higher doses should not be repeated too frequently**, especially 200c, 1m and 10m. These doses usually only need one to three initial doses to bring about a healing result.

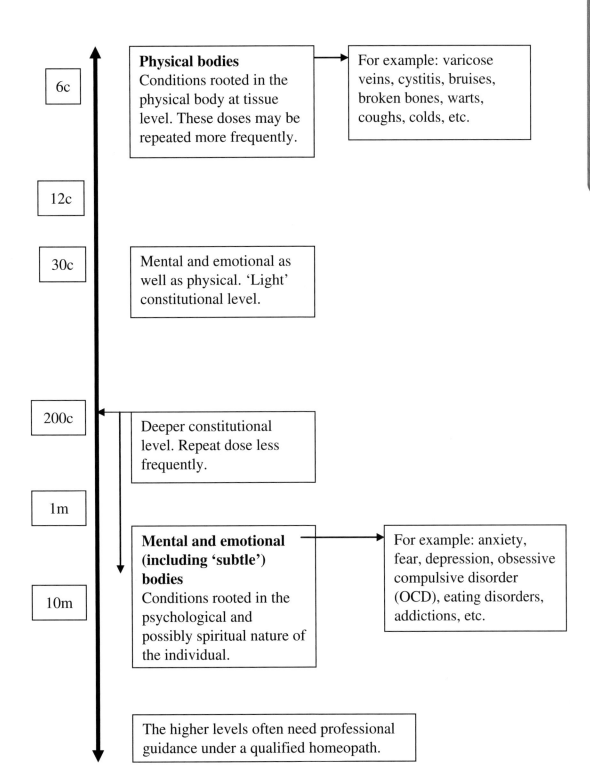

6c

12c

30c

200c

1m

10m

Physical bodies
Conditions rooted in the physical body at tissue level. These doses may be repeated more frequently.

For example: varicose veins, cystitis, bruises, broken bones, warts, coughs, colds, etc.

Mental and emotional as well as physical. 'Light' constitutional level.

Deeper constitutional level. Repeat dose less frequently.

Mental and emotional (including 'subtle') bodies
Conditions rooted in the psychological and possibly spiritual nature of the individual.

For example: anxiety, fear, depression, obsessive compulsive disorder (OCD), eating disorders, addictions, etc.

The higher levels often need professional guidance under a qualified homeopath.

Figure 5.1 The remedy doses

FAQs: Remedies

Do the remedies have to be stored in a particular way to increase their life span?
Yes. Remedies should be stored away from direct sunlight. Keep the lid securely fastened on the bottle or vial. Keep away from strong-smelling substances, such as perfumes, essential oils, household cleaners, toothpaste, mouthwashes, peppermints, and so on, as all these may have an antidotal effect on the remedy. The best way to store the remedies is in a homeopathic remedy storage box, available from all good homeopathic suppliers.

I went to a homeopath for treatment and they gave me a remedy to take, but I was not told what it was and there was no name on the bottle.
Some homeopaths do work in this manner, possibly because they do not want their patient to rush home and read all about the remedy and their personality type. Personally, I like my patients to know exactly what they are taking as this builds trust between homeopath and patient and also enhances the professionalism of the homeopath. I believe it is the patient's right to know the name and dose of the remedy they are taking, in the same way as is standard practice for all those prescribing allopathic (conventional) drugs.

a guide to treating common ailments

How to use this chapter

1 Look up your condition in the ailments section (listed alphabetically, below). Select one *or more* remedies that best match the key features of the ailment.

2 Check the selected remedy or remedies in Chapter 3: The remedies, to learn more about its modalities and characteristics. Does this still seem like the right remedy or remedies? Does it narrow down your selection if you had more than one remedy selected from step 1? You may still end up with more than one selected remedy that you feel is correct at this stage – this is acceptable.

3 Check if the selected remedy (or remedies) is one of the constitutional remedies as described in Chapter 2: The homeopathic constitutions; this may confirm your choice or highlight the one appropriate remedy if you still have more than one selected.

4 Make a final decision on the remedy. Keep a note of the other remedies that may have been selected in steps 1 and 2, but rejected because of step 3. These remedies may be needed if the first-choice remedy is ineffective.

5 Take the remedy in a dosage that is appropriate to the individual need (see Chapter 5: Taking the remedies and prescribing doses).

Acne

Description of condition

Acne is an inflammatory skin disease made evident by pimples that can appear on almost any part of the body, but usually on the face.

Other information

Topical use of Hypericum and Calendula tincture; use 20 drops (10 of each) in 0.25 to 0.5 pint of water, applied on a soaked cotton pad. May also need to be treated for stress.

Key features and remedies

Key features	Remedy
Spots that are slow to heal, may be almost boil-like.	HEPAR SULPH.
Sensitive individual. Very upset by appearance. Feels sad and weepy. Rich and fatty foods make it worse.	PULSATILLA
Skin may start to scar, especially if spots are picked or area is constantly touched. Skin is slow to clear and heal. Unhealthy look to skin. Low immune system.	SILICEA
Difficult to clear. Covers much of the face. Made worse by washing. Skin may look and feel rough.	SULPHUR

Agoraphobia

Description of condition

Fear of being in open places or situations from which escape might be difficult or embarrassing. Fear of being out of control or of losing control when in a public place (e.g. a restaurant or classroom). Fear of being in a place or situation in which help might not be available in the event of a panic attack.

Key features and remedies

Key features	Remedy
Individual becomes terrified, feels that they will faint or collapse.	ACONITE
Becomes cold, shivery and tired. Restless.	ARSEN. ALB.
Lacks will-power. Feels powerless. Suffocating feeling. Diarrhoea.	SULPHUR

Anorexia

Description of condition

Eating disorder. Denial of food, with fear of being overweight and a disturbed body image. Prevalent ages 10–25 years. More common in women than in men.

Key features and remedies

Key features	Remedy
Usually slim to start with. Complete loss of appetite. Aversion to food. Great fear of obesity, although never been overweight. Feels fatigued. May have twitches and shakes.	ALUMINA
Self-loathing and hate. Cannot bear own body image. Loss of appetite. Depression and lowness.	AURUM MET.
Loss of appetite. Wants salty foods when eating. Fixed ideas and fear of becoming overweight. Obsessive dieting. Grief for oneself, feelings of loss.	NAT. MUR.
Extreme under-nourishment. Weak immune system. Low self-worth that may stem from childhood.	SILICEA
Mind feels hurried. Rushed thoughts. Complete loss of appetite. Strong and fixed ideas about body image. Becomes very thin quickly. May suffer from verrucas and warts.	THUJA

Anxiety

Description of condition

A feeling of unease, apprehension or worry. It may be associated with physical symptoms, such as rapid heartbeat, feeling faint and trembling. It can be a normal reaction to stress or worry or it can sometimes be part of a bigger problem.

Key features and remedies

Key features	Remedy
Symptoms have a quick and sudden onset. Fear. Restlessness. Phobias. Nervousness. Sleeplessness. Shock. Palpitations.	ACONITE
Dread of known events. Overanxious, fear of failure. Fear of crowds. Vertigo.	ARGENT. NIT.
After shock or injury.	ARNICA

Oversensitive. Fear of being alone. Restless. Negative outlook. Obsessional, demanding, control freak.	ARSEN. ALB.
Timid and frightened. Jealous. PMS (premenstrual syndrome). Chronic fatigue syndrome.	CALC. CARB.
Anxiety from unhappiness and discontent with life.	CALC. PHOS.
Dread. Feelings of weakness and tiredness. Nervousness. Despondency. Panic. Sleeplessness. Fear of emotional breakdown.	KALI PHOS.
Constant talking. Jealous. Suspicious. Hypersensitive. Nightmares. Angry. Outbursts and temper tantrums. Hysterical. Fixed ideas. Chest may feel tight and constricted. Palpitations.	LACHESIS
Worry. Hair loss. Lack of confidence. Fear of being alone. Apprehensive. Chronic fatigue syndrome. Bottled-up fear. Stage fright. Confusion. Fear of a new situation.	LYCOPODIUM
Impatient. Irritable. Overindulgent. Prickly. Finds fault with everything. Argumentative. Angry. Critical. Hurried. Agitated. Short fuse. Temper. Sleeplessness.	NUX VOMICA
Anxious. Fearful. Does not like being alone. Hypersensitive. Stressed easily by external factors, such as storms, creeping insects, darkness. Fear is bottled up. Has fixed ideas. Fatigue. May suffer from twitches. Needs constant reassurance.	PHOSPHORUS
Tearful. Timid. Gentle. Obsessive compulsive behaviour (OCD). Fear. Changeable mood and symptoms. Likes to have sympathy.	PULSATILLA
Suppressed emotions and anger. Fear of loss of self-control. Workaholic.	STAPHISAGRIA

Backache

Description of condition

An aching sensation, often localized in the lower back, but can be reported elsewhere along the spine.

Key features and remedies

Key features	Remedy
Immediately after injury or strain. Feels or is bruised, as if from too much lifting.	ARNICA
Stiffness. Hurts with movement. Lower back pain with upper back stiffness (including the neck).	BRYONIA
Nerve pain. Coccyx injury. Inflammation. Sharp pain. May have sciatic pain.	HYPERICUM
Overexertion from activity (gym, gardening, etc.). Heaviness. Stiffness and pain. Tightness. Movement helps loosen the stiffness. Sciatic pain may also be present.	RHUS TOX.
Lower back and hip pain. Feels like deep pain. Sacroiliac pain. Referred pain to buttocks or top of thighs.	RUTA GRAV.
With period pain. Heaviness in legs. Feelings of sadness and despondency. Tearful and sensitive.	PULSATILLA

Other information

First stage of onset may be helped with Arnica in ointment, massage balm (in oil) or tincture (30 drops) used in the bath. Rhus Tox. can follow the Arnica as an ointment or massage balm (in oil), especially if injury is due to overexertion or general stiffness, or if sciatic pain is present. Ruta Grav. ointment is also useful if the feeling is of deep pain, hip pain, strained ligaments or tendons. A compress may also be used with Arnica tincture (20 drops to 0.5 pint of warm water).

Many homeopathic suppliers and pharmacies offer topical remedies combined (e.g. Arnica with birch and lavender; Arnica and Rhus Tox.; Hypericum with Calendula and chamomile – also excellent in an oil base for massage). All are of good therapeutic value, and it is worth having one as part of your first aid kit or to use as a regular back massage.

casestudy: Male (27 years), with back problems

A physiotherapist colleague, who was treating this patient's back, referred him to me. As a 'hands-on' therapist, I know how well homeopathy can work alongside this form of treatment. In my own career I started as a massage/sports therapist, then trained in aromatherapy and reflexology, as well as healing and, finally, homeopathy. In my own clinic I will often integrate these treatments, and with reflexology in particular, it is amazing how people open up and let go, telling you everything you need to know as a homeopath. This is an excellent approach for a client who finds it difficult to express their feelings. However, such an approach was not needed with this patient, as he was very open, friendly and positive.

He had worked as a landscape gardener for the past five years and was very proud of his work. A month before seeing me he had hurt his lower back while lifting. He thought it would improve over time without intervention, so took a few days off work. However, he found that he was still in pain when rising from a sitting position and when getting out of bed in the morning. He had visited his GP, who had sent him for an X-ray, which showed no major damage. Upon further discussion I also discovered that he did not want to take painkillers, as he thought they would upset his stomach and make the symptoms worse – this is an indicator of a Rhus Tox. personality type (fear of being poisoned by tablets). He had referred himself to a physiotherapist and had felt an improvement in his condition from the treatments (two treatments a week, with eight received to date). He had also been given stretches and exercises to complete at home. I felt that the home exercise aspect of the physiotherapy treatment was excellent, sharing responsibility for improving the condition with the patient, so that the patient plays an active part in the treatment and rehabilitation process – this is particularly important with back problems as there is often no quick fix for such symptoms. Many chiropractors and osteopaths also use the home exercise approach when treating their patients. His main purpose in seeing me was so that I could suggest homeopathic treatments that would help with his condition and thus prevent him from having to take the painkillers.

From the patient consultation I also learnt that he enjoyed exercise and keeping fit. He was a regular runner and went to the gym. He was physically strong and had to maintain his fitness level in order to be able to perform at work. He had not been troubled by major back problems in the past – just the occasional ache and pain that would disappear after a few days. There was no history of major accidents or illness. He was still working, but not lifting because of the current back problem. The physiotherapy was now once a week and he knew it would take time to fully recover, especially since he continued to work and thus put pressure on his back.

The symptoms were a sore, aching and bruised sensation around the affected areas, so Arnica was my first choice. Arnica is often called the healer, and most homeopaths think Arnica is best used at the first stages of an injury, accident or trauma, but it is worth noting that Arnica can help remove the trauma, shock and deep bruised feelings created by an accidental injury, strain or sprain, even if the event has occurred weeks, months or years before. Chronic problems that have arisen from a past injury may clear up successfully after treatment with Arnica. The mental aspect with Arnica can be a fear of being touched when in pain, and in this case the patient had sought help from his GP before having any hands-on treatment on his back, for fear of aggravating the condition. He did have a positive approach to his condition, however, referring himself to the physiotherapist very quickly after seeing the GP, and also believing that he would recover fully. These are also indicators of the Arnica personality, in that they report optimism and feeling well, even when ill, playing down their symptoms in an attempt to minimize their condition. This patient also reported feeling better for lying flat and worse from damp weather, both modalities that fit well with the Arnica type. Taking all this into account, I prescribed Arnica 30c in tablet form, to be taken twice a day for five days, and asked the patient to telephone me to book a further appointment. I also suggested taking an Arnica massage balm to his physiotherapy sessions so that he could ask for it to be applied on his back while the physiotherapist performed the massage and mobilizing treatment.

When we next spoke he said that after three days of taking the Arnica his back felt a little better, but that the symptoms had changed. The discomfort now appeared to be in the soft tissue and was sensitive to touch in the affected area. He reported this as feeling almost like the pain was working its way out from being a deep, aching pain to a more superficial bruising. I often refer to these reported changes as an 'inward to outward regression', in that the body will often exhibit a pattern of recovery, for example a downward regression from upper back pain to lower back ache, or an upward regression from shoulder to neck pain. The patient feels an improvement, but it is necessary to continue with the treatment, taking into account the signs given by the patient's own body in terms of the direction of the regression. I told the patient that his symptoms were an excellent sign that things were moving in the right direction and instructed him to reduce the Arnica to one tablet a day, after finishing work, until I met with him at his next appointment the following week.

When we next met he reported feeling much better, and that the physiotherapist was using the Arnica oil during the treatment and that he was applying it himself to the lower back before going to bed. He also said the sensitivity, which had increased, had now lessened, unless deep pressure was applied to his lumbar spine, although he also said that this pain triggered by deep pressure from the physiotherapist felt like 'good pain', in that it resulted in relief afterwards. I decided to stop the Arnica at this time as I did not want him to experience a proving of the remedy (i.e. develop symptoms that the remedy treats by taking it for too long). He also reported that the stiffness appeared greater on the right side and that he felt better for movement, as this seemed to free any feelings of stiffness, especially after a day at work. He reported that going for a brisk walk at lunchtime also helped mobilize his back and allowed him to continue working into the afternoon.

I suggested that the next remedy should be Rhus Tox., in a 30c potency, as this is ideal for aches and pains and for cases where the condition is better for movement and warmth. It is also indicated for conditions that are worse on the right side. As the patient was still reporting stiffness in the morning, I suggested taking one tablet on waking and one after work. One week later, at the next appointment, he reported feeling much better; his back was not as painful at the end of a working day, but still occasionally 'niggled' him during the day. He said that sleeping had improved, but that he still found himself waking in the night and having to change position to be comfortable. I commented that his mattress may need turning or replacing and that this could be contributing to the broken sleep and the stiffness first thing in the morning. I recommended a pressure-relieving mattress (e.g. the Tempur type) that would mould and support his body. I stressed that sleep was not only about rest, but also about regeneration and repair, and that a mattress was a good investment in his career as well as his body! I further recommended that the Rhus Tox. should now be only used when he felt overstretched, for example after a particularly heavy day of lifting at work – when the 'niggles' became obvious. In this case he should take a 30c tablet directly after work. This approach can also be used for strain or sprain immediately after any form of exercise. Rhus Tox. could also be used in a massage balm or oil when it was necessary to apply some relief directly to the affected areas. In terms of supporting products, I also mentioned that a supplement tablet of Glucosamine and Chondroitin Sulphate could be taken up to three times a day to protect and support the muscles, joints, cartilage and connective tissue. This supplement is excellent for promoting musculoskeletal support. I also suggested that

MSM Organic Sulphur would be useful, as it is an essential part of many body structures and enzymes, for example the proteins of connective tissue found throughout the body.

I believe it is vital to look at all the means available to help a patient prevent a reoccurrence of the presenting condition, as well as treating the actual condition itself. I often mention lifestyle advice and other natural remedies that may sit alongside the homeopathic treatment – but in cases of nutritional supplements I also stress that I am not a nutritionist, and that all supplements should be taken according to the directions on the label, and that if a patient is in any doubt about their suitability alongside existing medical conditions to consult their GP before taking the supplements.

I am pleased to report that this patient rang me a week after the final consultation to tell me that he had made a complete recovery, but that he was very aware that he needed to monitor and support his body with the homeopathic remedies and other treatments if there were any 'warning signs' of a reoccurrence. I was so pleased to hear that this patient was taking responsibility for the condition and listening to what his body was telling him. So often it happens that we ignore the symptoms, the condition worsens and we end up living around the condition rather than working towards its resolution. For example, a severe emotional upset can lead to anxiety, which can turn into depression, and this in turn affects how the body is held and can result in aches and pains, making for more depression – and so the circle continues. If the circle can be broken or the early problems treated, it follows that the more severe symptoms could be avoided and an earlier recovery made. Homeopathy affords the opportunity for a client to talk and be listened to; the homeopath can identify patterns of disease and behaviour towards the disease and draw strands of information together to identify early signs and symptoms, which can then be acted on with the appropriate remedies. Furthermore, remedies can be prescribed as a supportive treatment, so that even if a condition cannot be fully cured, it can delay or prevent completion of the circle.

On a final note, this patient telephoned again one month later to say that he wished he had shares in Arnica and Rhus Tox., as he had recommended it to several of his work colleagues, all of whom had reported beneficial effects! He wanted to thank me for my time and advice and to say that he would have no hesitation in recommending a homeopathic consultation to any of his associates and friends. I was so pleased that this patient had taken the time to make contact again – it makes all the difference to the homeopath to know a patient is still well after a month or more, as it helps with development of other patient cases and also makes the homeopath feel valued as a contributor to a person's optimum health.

Bad breath

Description of condition

Breath odour is unpleasant, distinctive or offensive. Severe cases can also be referred to as halitosis.

Key features and remedies

Key features	Remedy
Bad taste and smell in the mouth and feeling depressed.	AURUM MET.
Bad taste in the mouth, lots of saliva. Metallic taste in the mouth.	MERC. SOL.
After excess food and alcohol.	NUX VOMICA
With a dry mouth, often after eating certain foods (e.g. fatty foods).	PULSATILLA

Other information

Use mouthwash or gargle with natural-based products. Several homeopathic-based products are available.

Boils

Description of condition

Painful swellings of the skin caused by deep skin infection with bacteria. Boils begin as red, tender swellings, which may later ooze pus. Some people have recurrent boils. Individual boils can cluster together and form an interconnected network of boils called carbuncles. In severe cases, boils may develop to form abscesses.

Key features and remedies

Key features	Remedy
Skin feels very tight and hot over the boil. Needs cool application.	ARSENICUM
First stage when skin is tender and red. Throbbing and inflamed skin.	BELLADONNA
Very sensitive when touched. Slow to heal. May weep.	HEPAR SULPH.
Several boils that are slow to develop or slow to heal once the boil has burst.	SILICEA

Other information

Topical applications: can bathe or compress with Calendula or Hypericum tincture or a mixture of both (20 drops, 10 of each to 0.25 to 0.5 pint of water).

Bone breaks and fractures/ Common sprains and strains

Description of condition

There are many different names given to the types of broken bones and fractures suffered by the body (simple fracture, compound fracture, etc.), all of which refer to some form of damage to a bone or bones in the body. The bones provide a supportive and protecting function, as well as helping to enable movement. A sprain is a stretch and/or tear of a ligament. One or more ligaments can be injured at the same time. A strain is an injury to a muscle or a tendon.

Key features and remedies

Key features	Remedy
Sprains or strains with swelling or bruising. Sprains or strains with a bruised sensation. Immediately after breaks for shock and to aid healing of surrounding tissues.	ARNICA
Useful when bones are slow to heal. Individual feels tired and exhausted.	CALC. PHOS.
Strains that are swollen and painful, but better for gentle movement. For breaks after the cast is removed – to treat stiffness.	RHUS TOX.
Excellent for ankles and wrists, if symptoms are aching muscles and tendons.	RUTA GRAV.
Aids with bone healing.	SILICEA
For all bone injuries. This remedy will help the bone knit together, promoting healing and repair.	SYMPHYTUM

Other information

Arnica ointment for first stage of treatment (not on broken skin). Rhus Tox. ointment for second stage of treatment for stiffness. Ruta Grav. ointment also for second stage of treatment, particularly for ankles and wrists.

Bulimia

Description of condition

Eating disorder characterized by binge-eating, vomiting and purging, by vomiting or abusing laxatives.

Key features and remedies

Key features	Remedy
Much anxiety and fear. Binge-eating on sweets, chocolate, and so on.	ARGENT. NIT.
Feelings of slowness and exhaustion. Body feels congested and bloated. Large appetite. Suffers from constipation.	CALC. CARB.
Extreme hunger and appetite. Overweight. Feels low and emotionally drained. Feels guilty. Condition much worse when full of anxiety and nervousness.	GRAPHITES
Hypersensitive. Normally of slim build. Often creative or artistic. Increased appetite when stressed. Keeps condition hidden well and is fearful of others finding out.	PHOSPHORUS
Increased appetite in an overweight or plump individual. Emotions change from one minute to the next. Very emotional and weeps easily. Wants others to feel sorry for them. Enjoys sympathy.	PULSATILLA
Increased appetite in a dominant individual. Cannot sit still. Fidgeting, with poor posture and slouching. Binge-eating with fears of starvation.	SULPHUR

Catarrh

Description of condition

An inflammation of the mucous membranes, with a resulting free discharge of mucus. This affects the air passages of the head and throat and can be triggered by hay fever, rhinitis, influenza, bronchitis, pharyngitis and asthma.

a guide to treating common ailments

Key features and remedies

Key features	Remedy
Watery discharge. Burning feeling.	ARSEN. ALB.
Sore nasal passages. Yellow discharge.	CALC. CARB.
Pain, with a stuffy head cold.	NUX VOMICA
Chronic, sore nose. Bright blood on tissue when blown.	PHOSPHORUS
Yellow to green discharge.	PULSATILLA

Other information

Nasal sprays and/or drops are available containing homeopathic and other natural-based products.

Chickenpox

Description of condition

An acute, communicable, infectious disease, usually contracted by young children. Chickenpox is caused by the varicella zoster virus. The infection is characterized by a fever and itchy, red spots, usually appearing on the chest and stomach first, then in crops over the entire body. The red spots turn into small blisters that dry up and form scabs over about a week. They occasionally cause scarring (particularly if scratched) or if they become infected with bacteria.

Key features and remedies

Key features	Remedy
Quick, sudden onset, with first stages accompanied by anxious feelings and fearfulness. Thirsty.	ACONITE
Fever, with throbbing hot head and face. May have a headache.	BELLADONNA
Very sensitive and tearful. Especially children.	PULSATILLA
Restless and nervous. Many blisters in the first stages of the condition.	RHUS TOX. (also used as a preventative if in contact with chicken pox or shingles)

Chronic fatigue/Exhaustion/Post-viral syndrome/ME (myalgic encephalomyelitis)

Description of condition

A group of symptoms, of unknown cause, characterized by unexplained fatigue, weakness, muscle or joint pain, headaches, depression, feeling poorly, trouble thinking and sometimes fever and/or lymph node swelling. Post-viral syndrome (PVS) may follow a viral illness such as glandular fever.

Key features and remedies

Key features	Remedy
Total exhaustion, both mental and physical. Feels and looks old before their time. Weakness in muscles. Frustrated at being sick, wants a quick fix. Skin becomes dehydrated and dry.	ALUMINA
Slowness in mind and body. Feels down in the dumps. May develop sweats in the night. Feels fearful. Body feels congested.	CALC. CARB.
Poor memory. Exhaustion and fatigue. Loses interest easily. Feels unhappy with oneself.	CALC. PHOS.
Extreme exhaustion. Feeling emotionally and mentally weak.	CARBO VEG.
Onset after illness or infection. Feels sick. May have diarrhoea and night sweats. Headaches and tired eyes. Sensitive scalp. Irritable and difficulty in sleeping. Tired and weepy.	CHINA
Tiredness and exhaustion. Difficulty in expressing emotions. Very easily tired, yet strives to continue.	CUPRUM MET.
Symptoms come on after flu-like conditions. Anxious and fearful. Irritable. Hesitant to go out and socialize. Much fatigue. May feel dizzy when getting up in the morning.	KALI PHOS.
Professional, workaholic type. Feels exhausted. Worries about their condition. Digestive system may be affected (e.g. irritable bowel syndrome or IBS). Irritable state of mind.	LYCOPODIUM
Feels exhausted, depressed and run down. Weakness, with slight shaking or tremors. May have a sore throat and be prone to mouth ulcers and a bad taste in the mouth.	MERC. SOL.
Tired and weepy. Weak and does not want to be left alone. Light-headed when waking. Lethargic. Feels depressed and weighed down. Particularly useful for women.	SEPIA
Extreme tiredness and exhaustion. Down in the dumps and lowness of spirits. Becomes restless. Slowness of thought and mind. Sensitive and irritable. Memory becomes fuzzy and slow. Metallic taste in the mouth.	ZINC. MET.

Claustrophobia

Description of condition

An anxiety disorder that involves the fear of enclosed or confined spaces.

Key features and remedies

Key features	Remedy
Great fear and anxiousness. Fear of death.	ACONITE
Dread and fear. Loose bowels. Once in an open space recovers quickly.	ARGENT. NIT.
Becomes emotional. Cries and weeps easily.	PULSATILLA
Suffocating feeling. Feels powerless. Diarrhoea.	SULPHUR

Colds

Description of condition

A cold is caused by a virus infection located in the nose. Colds also involve the sinuses, ears and bronchial tubes. The symptoms of a common cold include sneezing, runny nose, nasal obstruction, sore or scratchy throat, cough, hoarseness and mild general symptoms, such as headache, feverishness, chilliness and not feeling well in general. Colds last for one week on average. Mild colds may last only two or three days, while severe colds may last for up to two weeks.

Key features and remedies

Key features	Remedy
Sudden onset. First stage of cold starts with not being able to sleep.	ACONITE
Watery eyes and sneezing.	ALLIUM
Flu-like symptoms. Chills and shivers. Aching limbs. Sore throat.	GELSEMIUM
Slow to clear in the last few days.	HEPAR SULPH.
Catarrh. Sneezing. Irritable. Chilly.	NUX VOMICA
With a hacking cough. Tight chest.	PHOSPHORUS
Heavy, aching limbs. Cold sore outbreak.	RHUS TOX.
Recurrent colds that are slow to heal.	SILICEA

Cold sores

Description of condition

Fluid-filled blisters, which appear as red, swollen areas of the skin or on the mucous membranes. The areas can be tender and painful. The blisters heal without scarring, but have a tendency to recur. Typically appearing on the face and lips, but also inside the mouth as blisters or small ulcerations. Cold sores are caused by a member of the herpes virus family, herpes simplex virus type one. It is caught through close contact (e.g. kissing) with someone who has a cold sore. You cannot catch cold sores from cups, flannels or towels. Many things trigger attacks: colds and flu, menstrual periods, emotional upset, fatigue, bright sunlight and cold winds.

Key features and remedies

Key features	Remedy
Sore, burning brought on by travel, sun and sea.	NAT. MUR.
First signs of blisters, with tingling and for chronic cases.	RHUS TOX.

Conjunctivitis

Description of condition

Inflammation of conjunctiva or membrane that covers the white of the eye and inner surfaces of the eyelid. Characterized by discharge, grittiness, redness and swelling. It may result from virus, bacteria, allergens, chemical exposure or ultraviolet light exposure and, depending on cause, can be contagious. Sometimes called pink eye.

Key features and remedies

Key features	Remedy
Sudden onset or after an injury.	ACONITE
Discharge. Blinking frequently. Watery.	ALLIUM
Swollen, burns and stings. Light sensitivity.	APIS MEL.
Yellow discharge. Styes.	PULSATILLA

Other information

Bathe eyes with Euphrasia tincture – use 20 drops to 0.5 pint of warm water. Use as an eye bath up to four times a day or soak on tissue pads to lie over eyes.

Constipation

Description of condition

A condition in which bowel movements happen less frequently than is normal for the particular individual, or the stool is small, hard and difficult or painful to pass.

Key features and remedies

Key features	Remedy
Much straining and dryness. Small stools. Hard and painful.	ALUMINA
Large bulky stool, hard and dry. Irritability. Painful, burning sensation.	BRYONIA
Bowels do not open for many days. Gripping pain when passed. Often very large stools.	GRAPHITES
Flatulence. Hard and painful stools. Movement occurs, but no stool is passed. IBS (irritable bowel syndrome), while pregnant and especially with travel.	LYCOPODIUM
Stools are dry, but light and often crumbly. Constipation every other day. Can feel like passing wind. Inactivity.	NAT. MUR.
From excess alcohol. Poor diet. Feeling cold and irritable. Need to pass stool, but can only manage small amount. 'Stuck' feeling.	NUX VOMICA

Cough

Description of condition

A sudden expulsion of air from the lungs that clears the air passages; it can be a symptom of upper respiratory infection or bronchitis; or as a result of an irritant.

Key features and remedies

Key features	Remedy
Sudden onset. Hard and constant cough.	ACONITE
Phlegm. Wheezy chest. Weak. Very tired. Hacking cough.	ARSEN. ALB.
Very dry, burning, with temperature. Feeling hot. Tickling and throbbing throat.	BELLADONNA
Very hard, dry cough. Spasmodic coughing. Sore chest. Headache. Body aches when coughing.	BRYONIA (also available as cough tincture)
Spasmodic cough that may bring on sickness or vomiting.	DROSERA
Bursting headache. Dry, hoarse throat. Hard cough. Irritable.	NUX VOMICA
Hacking, painful cough. Hoarse-sounding voice. Dry, tickling throat. Heaviness and tightness in chest.	PHOSPHORUS
Produces phlegm. Loose cough that dries up at night.	PULSATILLA
Bad taste in the mouth. Tired. Dry cough. May have catarrh. Excellent for cough during pregnancy.	SEPIA
Recurrent coughs that are slow to heal.	SILICEA

Cramp

Description of condition

A painful, involuntary, muscular contraction. Often there is no obvious cause, but it may occur with overexertion or chilling of the muscles. In most cases, the cramp goes away within a few minutes. Some common causes are muscle fatigue, heavy exercise, dehydration and pregnancy.

Key features and remedies

Key features	Remedy
With fatigue and exhaustion. From overexercise.	ARNICA
Mainly in legs and feet. First remedy of choice.	CUPRUM MET.
With a hangover or overindulgence of food. May also have headache.	NUX VOMICA

Other information

Arnica massage balm (in oil) can be massaged into the muscles.

Cystitis

Description of condition

A bladder infection marked by pain as well as frequent, painful urination.

Key features and remedies

Key features	Remedy
Burning and stinging when passing urine. Pain in lower abdomen. Attempt to urinate frequently. Little urine is passed.	APIS MEL.
Restless, chilly and anxious. Burning pain in lower abdomen. Feeling weak.	ARSEN. ALB.
Acute burning and throbbing sensation. Still feel need to pass urine after it has been passed. Dark urine. May have blood in urine.	BELLADONNA
Constant need to urinate. Cutting and burning sensation in abdomen. Little urine actually passed. Ache in lower back. Feelings of anger.	CANTHARIS
Constant burning sensation. After catheter. Develops after sexual intercourse.	STAPHISAGRIA
Need to urinate frequently, pain in bladder. After urination, feelings of tearfulness and sensitivity.	PULSATILLA

Other information

Hypericum tincture can be used in the bath to help with the infection (30 drops in the bath water).

Dandruff/itchy scalp

Description of condition

White flakes/scales in the hair due to excessive shedding of the scalp skin.

Key features and remedies

Key features	Remedy
Scalp with dry, scaly patches. Itchy and sensitive to touch.	ARSEN. ALB.
Dandruff with eczema or crusty patches.	GRAPHITES
Skin in scalp very dry. Greys early, many flakes. Hair that falls out.	LYCOPODIUM

Other information

Several topical-based products, Calendula or rosemary shampoo and conditioner. Hypericum and Calendula tincture as a final hair rinse (20 drops in a 0.5 pint of warm water).

Dental procedures – afterwards

Description of condition

Any form of intervention or support given by a dental professional to the mouth or gums.

Key features and remedies

Key features	Remedy
After procedures for shock and emotional upset, with much anxiousness.	ACONITE
First remedy after any form of treatment. Promotes healing, reducing swelling and bruising.	ARNICA
To help with healing of all teeth problems.	CALC. PHOS.
Pain and soreness after treatment and to prevent infection.	HYPERICUM
Puncture wound, after several injections or incisions.	LEDUM
Bleeding after treatment. Bright-red blood. Feeling hypersensitive.	PHOSPHORUS
After cuts and incisions.	STAPHISAGRIA

Dental procedures – before

Description of condition

Any form of intervention or support given by a dental professional to the mouth or gums.

Key features and remedies

Key features	Remedy
Excellent before procedures if nervous and anxious. Intense fear and tension.	ACONITE
Before and after the procedures to aid healing. Assist with blood clotting. Alleviate aching and bruising.	ARNICA
To prevent or treat infection and help heal wounds (i.e. gums).	HYPERICUM

91

Dental procedures – fear of

Description of condition

Anxiety or panic attacks resulting from the thought of undergoing dental procedures. Can also result in physical symptoms, such as palpitations, sweating and shaking.

Key features and remedies

Key features	Remedy
Great terror and fear, accompanied by disturbed sleep before the event.	ACONITE
Much sensitivity to pain and discomfort. Remedy of choice for a young child, especially with fear in the waiting room.	CHAMOMILLA
Weak and shaking. Trembling and very nervous.	GELSEMIUM

Depression

Description of condition

A mental state of depressed mood characterized by feelings of sadness, despair and discouragement. Depression ranges from normal feelings of 'lowness', through to major depression. There are also often feelings of low self-esteem, guilt and self-reproach, withdrawal from interpersonal contact and physical symptoms, such as eating and sleep disturbances.

Other information

Aurum Met./lavender and rose ointment can be applied to the heart area with gentle, clockwise massage movements using the fingertips. Apply morning and night for as long as needed. To balance and soothe the mind and body and to lift one's spirit and self-worth. To help centre the self.

Key features and remedies

Key features	Remedy
When restless. Constantly fussing and tidying things. Irritable and agitated. May pace around. Thinks nothing will help.	ARSEN. ALB.
Great onset of sadness, lowness, like a black cloud has descended. Low self-worth. Fed up and despondent.	AURUM MET.
Exhausted and slow. Weakness in thought and concentration. Feels sad and run down. Full of worry.	CALC. CARB.
Easily loses interest. Complains a lot. Discontented and unhappy with oneself and life.	CALC. PHOS.
Mind will not switch off. Sad and depressed. Feels physically drained from constant mental activity. Diarrhoea triggered by worry and stress.	CHINA
Very indecisive. Sadness and lowness makes a withdrawn and timid personality. Skin may be dry.	GRAPHITES
Depression with tiredness that may be triggered by surgery. Feelings of tightness in body and mind.	HYPERICUM
Much grief and sadness. Feels that they will never be happy. Following death of a loved one.	IGNATIA
Anxious and sad. Does not want to see people or socialize. May affect sleep and triggers nightmares.	KALI PHOS.
Sadness with great jealousy. Over-the-top reactions to events. Suspicious and talkative.	LACHESIS
Feelings of loss and grief for self. Does not want to talk about it. Great difficulty in letting go and moving on. After break-up of a relationship or loss or death of a loved one.	NAT. MUR.
Restless, irritable depression. Sudden onset. Self-critical. High achievers feel they have let themselves down.	NUX VOMICA
For highly strung, sensitive and creative individuals. May 'live on their nerves'. Constantly need approval and reassurance from others.	PHOSPHORUS
Low of spirit and weeps a lot. Changeable symptoms and mood. Bottled-up fear. Obsessive compulsive disorder. Can be prone to binge-eating and insomnia.	PULSATILLA
Extremely restless. Feelings of sadness and loneliness. Constantly on the go. Finds it difficult to stay still. Does not like taking pills. Strong fear of being poisoned from any medication.	RHUS TOX.
Sadness and generally feeling low. Lacks confidence. Feels heavy and weighed down. Only wants to do things they enjoy. Good remedy for women. Indifferent to loved ones. Tired and weak. Weeps easily. Postnatal depression.	SEPIA
Appears unable to express thoughts or emotions. Rapid mood changes. May become aggressive. Fear of the dark.	STRAMONIUM
Selfish individual. Dominant personality. No motivation when sad and low. Does not want to work. Post-menopausal depression. May become addicted to cigarettes or alcohol.	SULPHUR

Dermatitis

Description of condition

An inflammation of the skin caused by an allergic reaction or contact with an irritant. Typical symptoms of dermatitis include redness and itching.

Key features and remedies

Key features	Remedy
Mainly on the hands, between the fingers and toes. On or behind the ears. Skin can weep.	GRAPHITES
Dry, burning sensation and red in appearance. Reacts to heat and washing.	SULPHUR
In the last stages it is slow and hard to heal. May have been infected and is very sensitive.	HEPAR SULPH.
See-through blisters that itch and may weep. Hands and feet can be affected. In the last stages of healing the skin dries and peels.	RHUS TOX.

Other information

Graphites cream can be applied four times a day. It does not leave a greasy residue, so fits into a daily routine. The cream can be replaced with an ointment at night for a greater lubricating effect (not on the face). Especially good for the hands, feet and face (cream only should be applied to the face).

Calendula can be used at the first signs of dryness and sensitivity – this may help prevent further onset of the condition. Some suppliers offer combination creams and ointments containing several remedies; these are worth trying (e.g. Dermatodoron Ointment).

Remember, often skin problems can develop when we become stressed. In such cases, treat the stress with a remedy, before the skin has chance to react.

Diarrhoea

Description of condition

Frequent and watery bowel movements; can be a symptom of infection, food poisoning, colitis or, in rare cases, an intestinal tumour.

Key features and remedies

Key features	Remedy
From or with food. Feeling weak. May vomit.	ARSEN. ALB.
In babies and young children.	CHAMOMILLA
As above, but also accompanied by fever. Cold and shivery. Frightened.	GELSEMIUM
Caused by overeating and overindulgence. Irritable.	NUX VOMICA
Very sensitive. Fearful. Exhausted. Nervous.	PHOSPHORUS

Earache

Description of condition

Ear pain. An ache or pain arising in the ear. Medically it may also be called otalgia or otodynia.

Key features and remedies

Key features	Remedy
Very painful. Sudden onset. Feels hot.	ACONITE
Throbbing. Very hot, with hot face. Swollen glands.	BELLADONNA
Pain and discomfort, in particular with babies and children.	CHAMOMILLA
Slow to heal, starting with a sore throat.	HEPAR SULPH.
Blocked Eustachian tubes. Catarrh. General aching.	PULSATILLA

Other information

If prone to ear infections, regular treatment with natural-based ear drops, such as herbal aloe gold ear drops.

Eczema

Description of condition

An inflammation of the skin, usually causing itching and sometimes accompanied by crusting, scaling or blisters. Some types of eczema can be made worse by allergic reaction to wool, foods, skin lotions, and so on. Young children are often more prone to eczema.

Key features and remedies

Key features	Remedy
Honey-coloured discharge, can affect the face, eyelids, scalp, behind the ears and in the crease of the skin (elbows, back of knees, wrists, etc.).	GRAPHITES
Very dry skin that may crack.	PETROLEUM
Blister-like and itchy. May weep and then become dry. May look like skin is peeling as it heals. Often works well after other remedies, such as Graphites, have already been used, as it may complete the healing process.	RHUS TOX.
Itchy and dry skin. Feels rough and may burn. Washing aggravates.	SULPHUR
Extreme itching and burning. Inflamed and blotchy, like prickly heat or nettle rash. First reactive stage.	URTICA

Other information

Topical applications: Calendula cream can be used as a regular skin moisturizer, to help prevent skin conditions and in the first stages. Calendula oil can be used for regular body massage. Graphites cream is excellent for hands, face, scalp/hairline and behind the ears. In ointment form it can be used in skin creases, such as elbows and behind the knees. Urtica cream or ointment can be used for very itchy, dry skin caused by reaction to heat or when the skin is not weeping.

Some suppliers offer combination creams and ointments containing several remedies; these are worth trying (e.g. Dermatodoron Ointment). Hypericum/Calendula tincture mix of bath oil is good for a calming, soothing soak. Hypericum and Calendula tincture can also be used as a compress or hand soak if the skin is prone to infection (20 drops in 0.5 pint of water).

Remember, often skin problems can develop when we become stressed. In such cases, treat the stress with a remedy, before the skin has chance to react.

Exam nerves

Description of condition

Feelings of anxiety, stress and tension that may manifest themselves just before an examination, with physical symptoms such as twitching, palpitations, sweating and shaking.

Key features and remedies

Key features	Remedy
Extreme anxiety. Fear of failure. Cannot sleep the night before. May suffer palpitations.	ACONITE
Stress and tension. Dread builds up before the exam day. May get upset stomach and feel sick. Usually does well once sitting the exam, recovers quickly afterwards.	ARGENT. NIT.
Feels shaky and weak, almost fever-like. Very fearful.	GELSEMIUM
Much apprehension. Stomach feels like it is in spasm.	LYCOPODIUM
Feels run down. Suffers from mouth ulcers through stress. Headaches.	NAT. MUR.
Headaches through nervousness and too much study. Low self-confidence. Lacks assertiveness.	SILICEA
Feels exhausted, weak and drained. Poor memory.	ZINC. MET.

Extreme shyness

Description of condition

Fear of embarrassment in certain situations, such as at social events, when meeting new people or when speaking in public. In its extreme form, this is a type of social phobia, which can lead to alienation and depression.

Key features and remedies

Key features	Remedy
Much anxiety and panic. If made the centre of attention, then overcome by feelings of faintness.	ACONITE
Needs constant reassurance. Very hypersensitive. Fearful. Chest may become tight.	PHOSPHORUS
Very sensitive and quiet individual. Blushes easily and quickly. Can be easily embarrassed.	PULSATILLA

Flu

Description of condition

Acute viral infection of the respiratory tract caused by strains of the influenza virus. It is passed on by people breathing in liquid droplets containing the virus, which have been sneezed or coughed into the air. The symptoms, which include fever, headache, cough, sore throat and muscle aches, appear quickly.

Key features and remedies

Key features	Remedy
First stages that have a sudden onset accompanied by anxiousness and restlessness. Hot and cold feelings. Cannot sleep.	ACONITE
Tiredness and exhaustion. Stomach may also be upset. Sensitive. Feeling chilly and restless.	ARSEN. ALB.
High temperature. Burning and throbbing face and body. Eyes also hot and sore.	BELLADONNA
Pain from coughing. Dry throat, mouth and lips. Does not want to move about, pain throughout the body.	BRYONIA
Early stages where the body feels weak and tired. Aching, sore throat. Backache. Hot eyes and face. Temperature.	GELSEMIUM
With upset stomach. May feel run down by overindulgence of alcohol and food. Feels very cold, chilly and irritable just before onset.	NUX VOMICA
Body feels heavy, aching and stiff. Headache at the base of the skull. Dry cough.	RHUS TOX.

Other information

Arnica tincture (30 drops) can be used in the bath to relieve muscle aches and shivers. Arnica balm (oil) can also be rubbed on the back and limbs to help soothe aches and pains. Arnica and Rhus Tox. massage balm (oil) can be used for aching necks and backs. Several combination remedies are available in tablet or drop form. Cough tinctures are also available (e.g. Bryonia).

Food poisoning, upset stomach

Description of condition

Caused by consuming food contaminated with pathogenic bacteria, toxins, viruses, prions or parasites. Nausea, diarrhoea and headache are common indicators.

Key features and remedies

Key features	Remedy
Sickness with diarrhoea. Through eating bad food. Stomach feels painful and aching. Feels restless and cold.	ARSEN. ALB.
First remedy of choice. Sickness after eating. May also have a headache. Feels much better after vomiting.	NUX VOMICA

Glandular fever

Description of condition

An infection caused by a virus. It is also known as infectious mononucleosis, and even 'kissing disease' because of one of the ways in which it is passed on. Glandular fever can last for some months. It can affect any age group, from tiny babies to old people, although it is most common among teenagers. The initial infection causes symptoms which may include sore throat, fever, loss of appetite, tiredness and swollen glands. Sometimes the initial symptoms go unnoticed, but chronic lethargy sets in. Only then does the person become aware that something is wrong. Glandular fever can lead to chronic fatigue syndrome, which is sometimes called ME (myalgic encephalomyelitis). More serious problems may develop in glandular fever, including hepatitis (inflammation of the liver), haemolytic anaemia (where red blood cells are destroyed), encephalitis (inflammation of the brain), myocarditis (inflammation of the heart muscle) and neuropathy (nerve damage). Fortunately, these are rare and usually mild. An unusual reaction that sometimes alerts a doctor to the problem is a florid red rash, which can develop if someone with glandular fever is given penicillin.

Key features and remedies

Key features	Remedy
Sudden onset with fever. Face red and hot. Sore throat.	BELLADONNA
Heavy, aching feeling. Tired. Chills and flu-like symptoms.	GELSEMIUM
Sore throat, difficult to swallow – causing pain. Still wants to talk. Cannot tolerate anything around the throat.	LACHESIS
Limbs ache, stiff and heavy. Swollen glands and sore throat.	RHUS TOX.

Gum disease, gingivitis, sensitive teeth and gums

Description of condition

Gum disease is also called periodontal disease. It is the inflammation of the structures that surround and support the teeth. It is one of the most common causes of tooth loss. Gingivitis is inflammation of the gums, often caused by the long-term effects of plaque deposits.

Key features and remedies

Key features	Remedy
Sensitive gums and teeth. Bad breath. Metallic taste in the mouth.	MERC. SOL.
Swelling of gums. Bleeding gums. Prone to mouth ulcers or mouth ulcers already present.	NAT. MUR.
Very sensitive teeth. Gums bleed when brushing teeth. Bright-red blood.	PHOSPHORUS

Other information

Use mouthwash or gargle with natural-based product. Several homeopathic-based products are available.

Haemorrhoids/piles

Description of condition

Enlarged veins in the anus or rectum, generally caused by constipation or straining to have a bowel movement. Very common in pregnancy or after childbirth. An external haemorrhoid is outside the rectum; an internal haemorrhoid is inside the rectum. A prolapsed haemorrhoid is internal, protruding outside the rectum. A thrombosed haemorrhoid contains clotted blood.

Key features and remedies

Key features	Remedy
Sore, feeling bruised. Hotness. Throbbing.	HAMAMELIS
Sensitive, cutting and sharp. Bleeding.	HYPERICUM
With or from constipation.	NUX VOMICA

Other information

Some of the above remedies are available in creams and tinctures. Dietary factors can also influence – try to avoid alcohol and drink plenty of water. Hamamelis in a cream form is excellent to use up to four times a day and especially before bedtime.

Hair loss

Description of condition

The shedding of scalp hair. There are several types of hair loss, including male pattern baldness and alopecia.

Other information

Many natural-based shampoos and conditioners are available, such as rosemary-based products.

Key features and remedies

Key features	Remedy
After injury to the head or surgery.	ARNICA
Brought about by depression. Feelings of loneliness and despair.	AURUM MET.
After bereavement. Brought on by grief and emotional trauma.	IGNATIA
Early male pattern baldness. For women, after the birth of a child. May be associated with early greying.	LYCOPODIUM
With scalp problems, dandruff, and so on. Hairline may not be the first place to thin. Feelings of sadness and generally feeling low.	NAT. MUR.
Hair may fall out in clumps. Individual may be oversensitive.	PHOSPHORUS
Brought about by the menopause. Hormonal changes after childbirth.	SEPIA

Hangover

Description of condition

The after-effect following the consumption of large amounts of one drug or another. In particular, it is commonly associated with the overconsumption of alcohol.

Key features and remedies

Key features	Remedy
Overindulgence of alcohol. Feels terrible first thing in the morning. Head feels like it has been knocked or bruised.	NUX VOMICA

Hay fever

Description of condition

Hay fever is an allergic condition affecting the mucous membranes of the upper respiratory tract and the eyes. It is most often characterized by nasal discharge, sneezing and itchy, watery eyes. Hay fever is generally caused by an abnormal sensitivity to airborne pollen.

Other information

Homeopathic or natural-based sprays and nasal drops can also be used (e.g. Oleum Rhinale nasal drops or Rhinodoron spray – aloe-based).

Key features and remedies

Key features	Remedy
Sneezing. Very watery eyes. Sore nostrils.	ALLIUM
Itchy, ticklish nose. Painful when sneezing.	ARSEN. ALB.
Lots of sneezing. Burning eyes. Cough. Discharge.	EUPHRASIA (can also be given in spray and drop form)
Sneezing. Sore nose and eyes. Watery and itchy eyes.	MIXED POLLENS (before season – only available from homeopathic suppliers)
Constant sneezing. Nose running, then dry in the evening. Irritable.	NUX VOMICA

Headaches

Description of condition

Pain or discomfort in the head or face area. Headaches can be single or recurrent in nature, and localized to one or more areas of the head and face.

Key features and remedies

Key features	Remedy
Sudden onset. Anxious. Thirsty. Throbbing. Restlessness. Tightness. Pressure.	ACONITE
Stinging. Burning. Stabbing. Tender. Brain feels tired.	APIS MEL.
Weakness. Trembling. Eye strain through overconcentration.	ARGENT. NIT.
Bruised and aching. Sharpness.	ARNICA
Sharp, sensitive. Splitting and crushing. Feeling faint.	BRYONIA
Sharp headaches, concentrated in one spot. Mind constantly alert with thoughts and ideas. Hypersensitivity to pain.	COFFEA
Weak and shaky. Occipital pain. Heavy eyes. Blurred vision.	GELSEMIUM
Bursting, pressure headache. Tiredness and fatigue.	RUTA GRAV.
Builds up through anger. As if pressure needs to be released from the head.	STAPHISAGRIA
Irritable. Feels sick. Like a hangover.	NUX VOMICA

Incontinence/stress incontinence

Description of condition

The accidental or involuntary loss of urine or stool. A person may have urinary or faecal incontinence or both (sometimes called double incontinence). Stress incontinence is a condition in which urine leaks when a person coughs, sneezes, laughs, exercises, lifts heavy objects or does anything that puts pressure on the bladder, often due to weak muscles in the pelvic floor (can also occur during pregnancy).

Key features and remedies

Key features	Remedy
From coughing, sneezing and laughing. Walking can also trigger. Sometimes cannot feel leakage.	CAUSTICUM
Walking and during pregnancy. Need to pass urine increases when sitting or lying down. Flatulence and coughing.	PULSATILLA
'Bearing down' sensation from lower abdomen to vagina. Leakage while sleeping.	SEPIA

Indigestion

Description of condition

A disorder of the digestive function. Often characterized by discomfort, heartburn or nausea.

Key features and remedies

Key features	Remedy
Feels stressed and anxious. May also have diarrhoea and fluttering feelings in the stomach.	ARGENT. NIT.
With heartburn. Stomach feels heavy and weighed down. May feel sick and want to vomit. Feels tired yet restless.	ARSEN. ALB.
Bitter, dry taste in the mouth. Needs to drink cold fluids. Movement brings about sickness. Feels light-headed.	BRYONIA
Full of wind. Aching and burning sensation in stomach. Better after belching.	CARBO VEG.
Feels bloated, with wind. Tired and sluggish. May be worse after eating late at night.	CHINA
Stomach feels bloated and full. Heartburn. May also have IBS (irritable bowel syndrome). Constipation.	LYCOPODIUM
After too much food. With a hangover. Bad taste in the mouth.	NUX VOMICA
Hot, burning sensation in the chest. Tight chest. May bring on palpitations. Feels like a weight on the chest.	PHOSPHORUS
From foods too rich or fatty. Feels sick and wants to vomit. May have a headache. Feels emotionally upset, sensitive and weepy.	PULSATILLA
With sour taste in the mouth. Feels sick at the smell of food. Much flatulence and wind. Heavy, dragging feeling in stomach.	SEPIA

IBS (irritable bowel syndrome)

Description of condition

A disorder of the intestines that causes abdominal pain, which may or may not be accompanied by constipation, diarrhoea and/or bloating.

Key features and remedies

Key features	Remedy
Brought on by stress. Constricted wind, stomach ache. Constipation and diarrhoea. Tense and painful in the abdomen.	ARGENT. NIT.
Anxiety felt in the stomach. Aching in the stomach and bowels.	ARSEN. ALB.
Anxious. Tired and sluggish. Constipation. Still has good appetite.	CALC. CARB.
Burning sensation in the abdomen. Feelings of sickness. May vomit.	CANTHARIS
Exhaustion and low vitality. Weakness. Indigestion. Flatulence. General digestive disorders.	CARBO VEG.
Nervous feelings in the stomach. Exhaustion. Stress and oversensitivity.	KALI PHOS.
Bloated, constricted feeling around the bowels. Stomach pain.	LACHESIS
Feels full. Belching. Pain and discomfort in the bowel. Bloated. Spasms. Chronic fatigue.	LYCOPODIUM
Bloated and sensitive stomach after excess of food or alcohol. Abdominal cramps.	NUX VOMICA

Menopause

Description of condition

Menopause is a stage in life when a woman stops having her monthly period. By definition, a woman is menopausal after her periods have stopped for one year. Menopause typically occurs in a woman's late forties to early fifties. It is a normal part of aging, marking the end of a woman's reproductive years. Women who have their ovaries surgically removed undergo 'sudden' menopause.

Key features and remedies

Key features	Remedy
Dryness. Lack of vaginal lubrication. Feeling hot and flushed. Red face and throbbing feeling. Feeling hot, then feeling cold.	BELLADONNA
Dryness of skin. Lack of vaginal lubrication. Walls of the vagina become thin.	BRYONIA
Post-menopausal depression, with much indecisiveness.	GRAPHITES
Constricted feelings. Hot flushes. Sweating. Palpitations. Headaches. Very talkative. Heavy period. Post-menopausal depression.	LACHESIS
Hot flushes. Crying easily. Very sensitive. Prone to varicose veins and haemorrhoids.	PULSATILLA
Periods irregular. Hot sweats. A dragging and sinking feeling in the lower abdomen. Irritable. Menopausal depression, with slowness of thought. Weeps easily.	SEPIA

homeopathy in essence

Mouth ulcers

Description of condition

A mouth ulcer is a painful, open sore inside the mouth caused by a break in the mucous membrane. There are usually two main causes: accidental damage (e.g. overzealous brushing, minor burns from hot food and drinks, biting the inside of the mouth accidentally, a tooth that has become rough or orthodontic braces that rub against the gums); and an aphthous ulcer, which appears when someone is feeling stressed or under the weather. They often appear for the first time during puberty and can run in families. These mouth ulcers can take a couple of weeks to heal and more are likely to keep appearing until the individual is feeling relaxed and well again. Other, more serious, causes of mouth ulcers include herpes infection, inflammatory bowel disease and immune disorders, but these are usually accompanied by other symptoms around the body.

Other information

Use mouthwash or gargle with natural-based product. Several homeopathic-based products are available.

Key features and remedies

Key features	Remedy
Mouth is dry and burning. Ulcers are on the tongue and edge of the tongue. May have a bitter taste in the mouth.	ARSEN. ALB.
Ulcers may look yellow, with large ulcers on the tongue or at the bottom of the mouth generally. May also have bad breath.	MERC. SOL.
Ulcers in the mouth or on the tongue. Tongue may feel numb. Lower lip may be prone to dryness and cracking. Ulcers may be triggered by anxiety.	NAT. MUR.

Muscular aches and pains (including sports injuries and joint pain)

Description of condition

Muscle aches and pains are common and can involve more than one muscle at the same time. Muscle pain can also involve the soft tissues that surround muscles. These structures, which are often referred to as connective tissues, include ligaments, tendons and fasciae (thick bands of tendons).

Key features and remedies

Key features	Remedy
After a fall or injury. When strained or sprained. Feels bruised and muscles and joints ache.	ARNICA
Muscular and joint pain. Excellent for growing pains in children and teenagers – particularly in the legs.	DROSERA
Through overexertion or after sport. Stiffness in muscles and joints. Frozen shoulder. Stiffness improves with gentle movement.	RHUS TOX.
Deep aches and pains. Bone pain. Strained tendons and ligaments. Good remedy for elbows, wrists and ankles.	RUTA GRAV.

Other information

Arnica tincture can be used in the bath (30 drops in the bath water). Topical application of Arnica ointment is also useful. Ointments of Rhus Tox. and Ruta Grav. are also available. Massage oils with the above remedies will also help.

Nosebleeds

Description of condition

A nosebleed, medically known as epistaxis, is the relatively common occurrence of haemorrhage (bleeding) from the nose, usually noticed when it drains out through the nostrils.

Key features and remedies

Key features	Remedy
After injury and bruising.	ARNICA
Throbbing, with headache. Hot feeling on the face.	BELLADONNA
Bright-red blood. Regular bleeds. Very sensitive.	PHOSPHORUS

Operation – after

Description of condition

Any surgical procedure requiring local or general aneathstetic.

Key features and remedies

Key features	Remedy
Pain relief. Assist with clotting of blood. Prevents infection and aids healing. Bruising and swelling.	ARNICA
Aids convalescence.	CALC. PHOS.
Treat and heal infection. Also useful when depression is triggered after surgery.	HYPERICUM
Sickness from anaesthetic. Chest infections and tightness.	PHOSPHORUS
Promotes healing of cuts and incisions. Follows Arnica well.	STAPHISAGRIA

Operation – before

Description of condition

Any surgical procedure requiring local or general anaesthetic.

Key features and remedies

Key features	Remedy
Fear before an operation. Nervous and emotional stress and tension either days before or directly before the event.	ACONITE
To promote healing (take the day before an operation).	ARNICA
Weak and trembling with fear. Very apprehensive.	GELSEMIUM

Palpitations

Description of condition

A sensation that feels like the heart pounding or racing. The heart rhythm may be regular (normal) or irregular (abnormal). Some palpitations can also be felt in the chest, throat or neck.

Key features and remedies

Key features	Remedy
Sudden onset, with great fear and anxiety. Fear of death. Difficulty in getting to sleep.	ACONITE
Tight, constricted feeling in the chest and throat. Tightness in the chest, more on the left side. Worse when trying to sleep.	LACHESIS
Body tremors and shakes. Feels hot, with constrictions in the chest.	NAT. MUR.
After overindulgence, with hangover. After a heavy meal. Too much alcohol. Irritable.	NUX VOMICA
May be triggered from feeling too hot or after heavy, rich food. Feels weak and lethargic afterwards.	PULSATILLA

Other information

Aurum Met./lavender and rose ointment can be applied to the heart area, with gentle, clockwise massage movements using the fingertips. Apply morning and night for as long as needed. To balance and soothe the mind and body and to lift one's spirit and self-worth. To help centre the self. Will help to reduce fear.

Panic attacks

Description of condition

A period of intense fear or discomfort, typically with an abrupt onset. Symptoms can include trembling, shortness of breath, heart palpitations, sweating, nausea, dizziness, hyperventilation and sensations of choking or smothering. This condition is different from general anxiety because attacks are very sudden, appear to be unprovoked and are often disabling.

Key features and remedies

Key features	Remedy
Fear of death. Complete restlessness. Agitation and panic attacks, especially when waking from a nightmare.	ACONITE
Trembling with fear and feelings of total exhaustion.	GELSEMIUM
Extreme nervousness of people. Prone to hysteria.	KALI PHOS.
Fear and tightness in the chest. Dry throat. Voice becomes hoarse. Hypersensitive.	PHOSPHORUS

Other information

Aurum Met./lavender and rose ointment can be applied to the heart area, with gentle, clockwise massage movements using the fingertips. Apply morning and night for as long as needed. To balance and soothe the mind and body and to lift one's spirit and self-worth. To help centre the self. Will help to reduce fear and panic.

Premenstrual syndrome (PMS)

Description of condition

The physical and psychological symptoms that occur directly before (or in the week before) a woman's menstrual period. Symptoms may include bloating, headache, irritability, anxiety or depression, low self-esteem, difficulty sleeping, changes in appetite, fatigue and breast swelling and tenderness.

Key features and remedies

Key features	Remedy
Feeling heavy and bloated. Feeling low in spirit. Breasts may be tender.	CALC. CARB.
With jealousy and spitefulness. Suspicious. Feelings of nervousness and being on edge – especially when waking in the morning. Fluid retention. Anger.	LACHESIS
Bad temper. Lethargy. Depression and withdrawn state. Suited to intellectual types.	LYCOPODIUM
Feeling of grief and loss. Sadness. Fluid retention.	NAT. MUR.
Impatient and irritable. Constipated. Prone to lash out at others, especially just after period.	NUX VOMICA
Bursts into tears easily. Irregular periods. Changeable mood. Sore breasts.	PULSATILLA
Indifferent. Sadness and crying when alone. Depressed and feeling low. Irritable.	SEPIA

Raynaud's disease

Description of condition

The blood supply to the extremities – usually the fingers and toes, but sometimes also the ears and nose – is interrupted. During an attack the extremities first become white and dead-looking, then red and burning. There may be considerable pain, numbness or tingling.

Key features and remedies

Key features	Remedy
Skin feels swollen, itchy and tight.	ARSEN. ALB.
Very cold, mottled appearance to skin.	CARBO VEG.
Coldness and tingling. Blue colour to skin. Feels restless. Fingers and toes feel constricted.	LACHESIS

Other information

'Frost' cream is a homeopathic and natural-based combination remedy to improve peripheral circulation to fingers and toes. Massage the cream into the fingers and toes morning and night (also excellent for chilblains).

Restless legs

Description of condition

Feeling of uneasiness and restlessness in the legs after going to bed (sometimes causing insomnia); may be relieved temporarily by walking or moving the legs. Thought to be caused by a disorder of the nervous system that affects sensation and movement in the legs and causes the limbs to feel uncomfortable.

Key features and remedies

Key features	Remedy
Legs always twitching and moving. Great restlessness and anxiety.	ARSEN. ALB.
Worse when trying to sleep. Legs may throb and feel hot. Legs may spasm.	BELLADONNA
Muscle spasms in legs. May develop cramp at night. Feels tired and exhausted in the morning.	CUPRUM MET.
Broken sleep pattern because legs moving around. Much movement in the night. May be worse with loss or grief.	IGNATIA
Right side more affected. Legs are trembling.	PHOSPHORUS
Worse during the daytime. May feel heavy, with a dragging sensation.	SEPIA
Restless trembling. Twitching when sleeping. Feels exhausted even on waking. Tired and weak.	ZINC. MET.

RSI (repetitive strain injury)

Description of condition

A term used to refer to various kinds of work-related musculoskeletal injuries, such as carpal tunnel syndrome, tendonitis and bursitis. Such injuries are also known as cumulative trauma disorders (CTDs), work-related upper limb disorders (WRULDs) and occupational overuse injuries.

Other information

Topical application of Arnica, Rhus Tox. or Ruta Grav. ointment will help support the homeopathic treatment and relieve discomfort from the affected area.

Key features and remedies

Key features	Remedy
First signs of condition, with aching and bruised sensations.	ARNICA
Made much worse by any movement or when writing, typing and so on.	BRYONIA
Inflammation and nerve pain.	HYPERICUM
Feels stiff, painful, heavy and aching. Improves with gentle movement and stretching. Good remedy after Arnica.	RHUS T.UX.
Deep aching pain, like bone pain. Worse at the wrist. Feels weak.	RUTA GRAV.

SAD (seasonal affective disorder)

Description of condition

SAD is a depression that occurs each year at the same time, usually starting in autumn or winter and ending in spring or early summer.

Other information

When selecting a remedy for this condition, it is particularly worth applying the constitutional approach, especially if the listed remedies seem ineffective. Try waking up to a light-box alarm clock or eating your breakfast in front of a light box before starting your day. The light box has proved to be of benefit to many SAD suffers, due to its particular spectrum of light.

Key features and remedies

Key features	Remedy
Feeling low in winter months. Emotionally low, giving rise to extreme unhappiness and depression.	AURUM MET.
Exhaustion and fatigue, particularly in the winter months. Insecurity and unhappiness, when season changes to winter.	MERC. SOL.

Sciatica

Description of condition

Caused by pressure on the sciatic nerve, which passes through the pelvis. Symptoms include pain, tingling or numbness in the lower back and down the legs, and can last only a few hours, but may also be recurring or permanent. Often experienced due to strenuous activity or during pregnancy.

Key features and remedies

Key features	Remedy
Radiating pain down the buttocks and legs. Stiffness in the lower back.	RHUS TOX.
Pain from lower back, down the hip and upper leg.	RUTA GRAV.
Sharp, radiating pain, due to accident or injury.	HYPERICUM

Sinusitis (nasal pain)

Description of condition

An inflammation of the sinuses (hollow spaces in the bones of the cheeks and forehead), due to infection or an allergic reaction. Common symptoms of sinusitis include pain in the face, coloured (not white or clear) secretions from the nose and headache.

Other information

Nasal sprays and/or drops are available containing homeopathic and other natural-based products.

Key features and remedies

Key features	Remedy
Sudden discomfort and pain.	ACONITE
Catarrh. Nose bleeds bright-red when blown. Sneezing.	PHOSPHORUS
Blocked nostrils. Pressure pain.	PULSATILLA
Bones of face feel sore and sensitive.	SILICEA

Sleeplessness/insomnia

Description of condition

Sleep problems characterized by difficulty falling asleep, frequent waking during the night or waking up earlier than desired. Insomnia can result in getting up in the morning feeling unrested and experiencing drowsiness during the day.

Key features and remedies

Key features	Remedy
Great restlessness. Pain. Fear of not being able to sleep. After bad news, shock. When sleeping, often suffers from nightmares.	ACONITE
Feels heavy and aching all over. May have back pain, cannot get comfortable in bed.	ARNICA
Very apprehensive. Restless. Wakes up in the early hours.	ARSEN. ALB.
Cannot sleep through depression. Feelings of isolation and loneliness. Cannot see the bright side.	AURUM MET.
A child that is too active to sleep. May sleep if comforted and held.	CHAMOMILLA
Mind becomes very overactive. Cannot switch off or clear mind of worrying thoughts.	COFFEA
Cannot sleep through grief, loss or emotional upset. May have recurring nightmares.	IGNATIA
Overactive mind. Cannot relax from the day's work. Constantly waking from sleep.	LYCOPODIUM
Through overindulgence. Eating or drinking too much, particularly rich and spicy foods. Under a lot of mental strain.	NUX VOMICA
Wakes with restless thoughts. Feels hot and cold. Oversensitive and weepy.	PULSATILLA
Wakes up with stiffness in the joints. Aches and pains mean cannot get comfortable.	RHUS TOX.

Other information

Avena sativa comp. drops are a homeopathic and natural-based combination. Take 20 drops in half a glass of water, 20–30 minutes before sleeping, Use for up to one month to break the insomnia pattern and introduce restful sleep. Further doses can be taken if the insomnia returns.

Sore throat

Description of condition

Also known as pharyngitis, it is a painful inflammation of the pharynx. Infection of the tonsils, or tonsillitis, may occur at the same time.

Key features and remedies

Key features	Remedy (some available as gargles)
Sudden onset. Very painful to swallow. Dry feeling.	ACONITE
Stinging, burning. Swollen throat.	APIS MEL.
Throbbing, burning. Red and inflamed.	BELLADONNA
Shivers, flu-like symptoms. Very sore to swallow.	GELSEMIUM
Slow to heal.	HEPAR SULPH.
Painful with constriction. Sensitive to touch. Tight sensation.	LACHESIS
Ulcers in throat. Painful. Bad breath and bad taste in mouth.	MERC. SOL.
Sore, throbbing throat that is slow to heal.	SILICEA

Sore throat and tonsillitis

Description of condition

Inflammation or swelling of the tonsils. This swelling is usually caused by either a viral or bacterial infection.

Key features and remedies

Key features	Remedy
Sudden onset, dry and burning. Sensitive and sore when swallowing.	ACONITE
Throbbing, very painful throat. Tonsils red and swollen. May also have fever.	BELLADONNA
Tonsils and throat look infected and are slow to heal. May feel shivery, with a temperature. Sharp pain when swallowing. Glands in the neck are swollen.	NAT. MUR.
Swollen tonsils. Uncomfortable to swallow fluids. Feels tight and constricted around the throat.	LACHESIS
Ulcerated tonsils. Bad taste in the mouth. Metallic taste in the mouth. Mouth is stinging and sore.	MERC. SOL.
Recurrent sore, throbbing throat/tonsillitis that is slow to heal.	SILICEA

Teeth grinding

Description of condition

Also known as bruxism. The teeth are ground together or the jaw clenched tightly during sleep. Bruxism can be mild and occasional or can be so frequent and/or violent that the teeth are damaged. The cause in some cases is abnormal dental occlusion (the way the upper and lower teeth fit together when the mouth is shut). More often, the disorder is associated with anxiety, tension and suppressed anger.

Key features and remedies

Key features	Remedy
Restlessness, with grinding of teeth at night.	ARSEN. ALB.
First stages, grinding through stress and anxiousness. Cannot switch off at night.	ACONITE
Teeth may become loose or displaced. Feels exhausted and tired, even after waking in the morning.	ZINC. MET.

Other information

Avena sativa comp. drops are a homeopathic and natural-based combination. Take 20 drops in half a glass of water, 20–30 minutes before sleeping, to induce a deeper sleep, relaxation of jaw muscles and to encourage a regular, healthy sleep pattern. Use for up to one month or when feeling tense.

Tinnitus

Description of condition

Sensation of a ringing, roaring or buzzing sound in the ears or head, often associated with various forms of hearing impairment.

Key features and remedies

Key features	Remedy
Sudden onset by loud noise, such as music or drilling.	ACONITE
Continued hissing and buzzing sound in the ear, not disappearing after onset.	CHINA

Tooth abscess

Description of condition

A tooth abscess is a bacterial infection of the centre of a tooth. It is a complication of tooth decay. It may also result from trauma to the tooth, such as when a tooth is broken or chipped. Openings in the tooth enamel allow bacteria to infect the centre of the tooth (the pulp). Infection may spread out from the root of the tooth and to the bones supporting the tooth.

Other information

Tincture of Hypericum and Calendula for pain and infection. Promotes healing. Use the tincture as a mouth rinse, five to six drops in 0.5 pint of warm water up to three times a day, especially at night and after dental treatment.

Key features and remedies

Key features	Remedy
First stages of abscess. Area around site feels hot and throbbing.	BELLADONNA
Slow to heal after dental treatment.	HEPAR SULPH.
Metallic taste in mouth. Gum around the abscess feels swollen and spongy. Much saliva in the mouth.	MERC. SOL.
Very painful, swollen and angry. Difficulty eating.	SILICEA

Travel/motion sickness

Description of condition

Travel sickness, or motion sickness, occurs when your sense of balance (equilibrium) is temporarily upset. Certain motions cause the brain to receive mixed signals, which upsets the delicate balance mechanism of the inner ear and causes the brain to become confused. This results in feelings of nausea, vomiting and sweating.

Key features and remedies

Key features	Remedy
With jet lag.	ARSEN. ALB.
Constantly feeling sick. General travel sickness. Still feels sick, even after vomiting. Any form of motion makes the condition worse.	IPECAC.
Like a hangover, with feelings of sickness. Vomiting. Headache.	NUX VOMICA
When pregnant and sensitive.	PULSATILLA

Varicocele

Description of condition

A mass of enlarged veins that develops in the spermatic cord, which leads from the testicles (testes) up through a passageway in the lower abdominal wall (systeminguinal canal) to the circulatory system. The valves that regulate blood flow from these veins become defective; blood does not circulate out of the testicles efficiently, which causes swelling in the veins above and behind the testicles.

Key features and remedies

Key features	Remedy
Heavy, aching feeling, with burning sensation.	HAMAMELIS
Left testicle affected. Feels swollen, tight and constricted, with aching.	LACHESIS
Feels heavy and aching. Needs support (briefs instead of boxers).	PULSATILLA

Varicose veins

Description of condition

Enlarged, twisted, painful, superficial veins, resulting from poorly functioning valves. Seen most often in the legs (also called varicosities), although they can be found in other parts of the body. Usually they appear as lumpy, winding vessels, just below the surface of the skin. There are three types of veins: superficial veins that are just beneath the surface of the skin; deep veins that are large blood vessels found deep inside the muscles; and perforator veins that connect the superficial veins to the deep veins. The superficial veins are the blood vessels most frequently affected by this condition and are the veins that are visible when the varicose condition has developed.

Key features and remedies

Key features	Remedy
Heavy and aching legs. Skin looks mottled. Poor circulation.	CARBO VEG.
First remedy of choice when veins first appear. Legs feel heavy, aching, bruised and sore.	HAMAMELIS
Burning, stinging and aching feeling. Legs feel constricted. A need to wear loose clothing. Left leg is worse than the right.	LACHESIS
During pregnancy. Individual may be sensitive. Legs feel heavy and aching.	PULSATILLA
Feels weak and exhausted.	ZINC. MET.

Other information

Topical applications of gel and creams containing Hamamelis or a combination of several remedies. Many different products available.

casestudy: Female (46 years), with varicose veins

A friend of this patient, whom I had treated, had recommended homeopathic treatment. The patient was fair-haired, of medium build, with a gentle, sensitive and caring manner. Her presenting condition was varicose veins. The varicosities were affecting both legs, although worse on the right leg. There was also swelling present around both ankles. After the initial consultation it was evident that she was in good emotional and physical health, apart from the varicose veins. She did admit to being oversensitive – she gave an example that if one of her three children became unwell she would 'feel the pain' herself. This put me in mind of a Pulsatilla personality type. When relaxing she would lie back and put her hands behind her head – again, this is a strong indication of the Pulsatilla type.

She worked four days a week in a large department store, which involved constant standing, and since leaving school she had worked in other jobs of this type, which involved long periods of standing. On a practical note, I suggested never using the escalators in the store where she worked, but to take the stairs whenever she could, to provide some exercise and stimulation to the legs and to help pump the blood and lymph to ease the aching legs. I also suggested support tights, and was amazed when she said she had not worn any – especially knowing that they would have helped. I also mentioned that resting the legs in an upright position when at home would also be of benefit. She reported that the veins had gradually got worse after giving birth to her three children. She was fearful of an operation to help remove the veins, although I did explain that there were many new treatment options available and that it may not be necessary to endure a 'stripping' operation.

My first thought was towards Pulsatilla, but as the veins did not feel worse when they were hanging down (e.g. sitting on a barstool), I needed a remedy that would match the symptoms of burning, stinging, swelling and a feeling of heat in the legs, along with general discomfort most of the time, particularly while standing, with some movement. I decided upon Hamamelis, in 6c potency. I prescribed one tablet three times a day until some relief was felt. Hamamelis is excellent in helping the symptoms associated with this condition. While the remedy will not repair the varicose veins once the valves have malfunctioned and the elasticity in the vein wall has become weak, it will have a toning effect on the veins, helping prevent further damage. I suggested a week of this remedy before the support tights were used, so we could monitor its effectiveness. I also recommended a topical application of Arnica with witch hazel (skin tone lotion produced by Weleda), as this is a gel that can be applied in the morning, before putting on tights, and reapplied at lunchtime, as it does not produce a sticky effect. It is best used cold, straight from the fridge, in order to have an astringent effect. It can also be used at the end of the day. The topical application would complement the remedy and make the legs feel less hot, heavy and aching. It also keeps the skin in good condition, as varicose veins can often be a precursor to dry and discoloured skin, which can result in varicose eczema. If eczema was already present I would have suggested Graphites cream as an additional application to the affected areas. The Arnica and witch hazel would also help to alleviate any swelling of the ankles caused by fluid retention.

I saw her again 10 days later and was pleased to note that although she still reported the legs as aching, she also felt that it was not as obvious. In fact she thought it was about 50 per cent improved, as much of the stinging and burning had subsided. I suggested that she now begin to wear the support tights, and that it was important to get the pharmacist to measure her for them, as having the right size and fit was very important. I asked her to continue with the Hamamelis, but to lower the dose over the next week to one tablet twice a day. When we next spoke on the telephone she reported an 80 per cent improvement, and that she was following all the advice – using the tablets, gel and support tights. I felt that, as this was a longstanding condition, we had reached as much of an improvement as we could expect, so I suggested continuing with the gel three times a day, and using the Hamamelis 6c twice a day, but only on the days she was working. I hoped this would maintain the improvement in her condition. I also discussed with her that if any further complications arose (e.g. a worsening of the symptoms or the appearance of new symptoms), to contact me again. This patient shows how the remedies can fit well into a daily routine, and can be used alongside other complementing treatments.

Warts

Description of condition

Warts are skin growths caused by a virus. They have a rough surface on which tiny, dark specks may be seen. They may grow on any part of the body and their appearance depends on their location. They are generally harmless, although in rare cases it may indicate more serious skin and viral problems.

Key features and remedies

Key features	Remedy
For all types of warts, cauliflower-type warts on the hands and face and flat warts on the feet, including verrucas.	THUJA
Mainly on the face or fingertips. Sore and painful verruca.	CAUSTICUM
Warts and verrucas that burn and sting or ache and feel hard.	SULPHUR

Other information

Topical applications: Thuja tincture can be applied two to three times a day, especially after bathing or washing. The cream can be used on the face, but not near the eyes.

FAQs: Homeopathic treatment

How do I find the right practitioner for me?
Always check the practitioner holds a qualification in homeopathic medicine. Use a list of practitioners supplied by a homeopathic organization or society. Also ask around for a recommendation through friends, your family doctor or health food store; as well as looking for a qualified homeopath, it is always advisable to use one who has been recommended by others. An excellent list of academic qualifications does not, in itself, make an excellent practitioner. When visiting a homeopath, look for their knowledge of the remedies and their ability to use intuition and their social interaction skills, to understand your condition and treat you in a non-judgemental and respectful manner. Word of mouth is always the most reliable way to find a good homeopath – you will often hear the same name being recommended by several people, which is always a good sign.

Can I try a few different therapies and supplements to help to improve my condition? My last therapist said I should have only one thing at a time.
It is important that the patient follows what feels right for them. The only reason to avoid other therapies would be if substances were being used that would counteract the homeopathic remedies. My opinion is that the primary concern of any therapist should be to get the patient well, irrespective of what makes them well. We need to remove the ego from the practitioner and to celebrate a patient's improved condition, whether this is due to a practitioner with a weekend's training in healing or one with four years' full-time study in osteopathy; whether qualified for five minutes or five years – the point is *the patient got well!*

Can I get homeopathic treatment on the NHS?
Yes. It is possible to be referred to a homeopathic hospital by your doctor, or treated directly by your doctor if they have been trained as a homeopath and are offering homeopathy within their practice.

I have tried a remedy and received no benefit from it – does this mean homeopathy will not work for me?
Sometimes it is necessary to try several remedies before we find the one that will work best. It is important to report back to your homeopath if a remedy is having no effect after several days, so that a different remedy can be tried. For example, taking

Lycopodium for IBS may result in no positive improvement, so Kali Phos. may be tried instead. The remedy choice may be varied to take into account the different personality types or changes in external circumstances that may affect the condition (e.g. stress and exhaustion). The remedy may be changed yet again to Nux Vomica if the symptoms are made worse by an excess of rich food and alcohol. If the stomach feels bloated, tight and constricted, with a need to wear loose clothing around the affected area, the remedy choice may be Lachesis. In this way, the constitutional aspect of a remedy may dictate changes in the prescription pattern.

Can homeopathy work on my pet?
Yes it can. There are several books on homeopathy for animals, including treatments for cats and dogs. There are also qualified vets who have taken courses in homeopathy. Always consult a qualified vet before giving any remedies to animals.

How long can I take a homeopathic remedy for?
For self-prescribing it is usual to take the remedy for three to four days. It can take longer for the effects to be felt in cases where the condition has been present for a long period, as is often the case with varicose veins or depression, for example. It is important to state that every individual is unique and will respond differently, so the dosage always depends on the reaction to treatment. It is never the same for everyone, as is befitting of a holistic therapy.

7 chapter

stress and homeopathy

Stress factors

Each of us carries the potential to contract disease at any time. However, only certain people become ill, while others stay healthy. It is the mental and physical condition of the body that causes subtle changes in hormonal and defence mechanisms, thereby allowing the disease or virus to manifest. By treating the whole person, with the holistic approach, we enable equilibrium, or homeostasis, to be restored, where circulation can flow unimpeded and supply nutrients and oxygen to the cells. The body's organs (which are no more than a collection of cells) may then return to a normal state of function.

It is generally accepted that 75 per cent of all disease is caused by stress. However, a certain amount of stress is needed for us to function; it is only when this becomes too much that disease can result. Everyone has different tolerance levels. It can help to view stress like a temperature gauge, in that it encompasses a wide set of values, and these values reflect perceptions of 'good' and 'bad'. For some a

low temperature is intolerable and therefore bad, while for others it is preferable, and good. Others still may adapt and grow used to it.

A useful definition for stress when it becomes a problem is: **the body's reaction to events and emotions that seem to be outside its conscious control or give a feeling of an inability to cope.** From this definition we can see that each person will have a different perception of their own stress levels.

The homeopath should be alert to stress factors in a client and indications that the client's coping mechanisms are under undue strain. This information will be gathered during the initial consultations, from the treatments process and from interaction with the client during the treatment process. From this information a prescribing remedy can be selected. The table below (page 127) gives some key features when considering stress-based remedies.

As well as taking a homeopathic remedy, a stressed client needs to become aware of their own triggers for the condition. This awareness may only become apparent once a client has begun to take their selected remedy, as the remedy may in itself prove to be a catalyst for a client's examination of their own stress factors. When a client becomes more aware of their triggers, it becomes possible to examine the reasons for these and develop coping strategies.

Hans Selye

Dr Hans Selye (1907–82) was born in Vienna. As early as his second year of medical school (1926) he began developing his now famous theory of the influence of stress on people's ability to cope with and adapt to the pressures of injury and disease. He discovered that patients with a variety of ailments manifested many similar symptoms, which he ultimately attributed to their bodies' efforts to respond to the stresses of being ill. He called this collection of symptoms 'this separate stress disease', 'stress syndrome' or 'the general adaptation syndrome' (GAS).

He spent a lifetime in continuing research on GAS and wrote some 30 books and more than 1500 articles on stress and related problems, including *Stress without Distress* (1974) and *The Stress of Life* (1956). So impressive have his findings and theories been that some authorities refer to him as the Einstein of medicine.

A physician and endocrinologist with many honorary degrees for his pioneering contributions to science, Selye also served as a professor and director of the Institute of Experimental Medicine and Surgery at the University of Montreal. More than anyone else, Selye has demonstrated the role of emotional responses in causing or combating much of the wear and tear experienced by human beings throughout their lives. He died in 1982 in Montreal, where he had spent 50 years studying the causes and consequences of stress.

In his paper 'The nature of stress', Selye presented some excellent overriding principles that he felt could be used to counteract the undue stress felt by certain individuals. He wrote in this paper that 'after four decades of clinical and laboratory research', he could summarize the most important principles as follows:

■ Find your own stress level – the speed at which you can run toward your own goal. Make sure that both the stress level and the goal are really your own, and not imposed upon you by society, for only you yourself can know what you want and how fast you can accomplish it. There is no point in forcing a turtle to run like a racehorse or in preventing a racehorse from running faster than a turtle because of some 'moral obligation'. The same is true of people.

■ Be an altruistic egoist. Do not try to suppress the natural instinct of all living beings to look after themselves first. Yet the wish to be of some use, to do some good to others, is also natural. We are social beings, and everybody wants somehow to earn respect and gratitude. You must be useful to others. This gives you the greatest degree of safety, because no one wishes to destroy a person who is useful.

- Earn thy neighbour's love. This is a contemporary modification of the maxim 'Love thy neighbour as thyself.' It recognizes that not all neighbours are lovable and that it is impossible to love on command.

Perhaps two short lines can encapsulate what I have discovered from all my thought and research:

Fight for your highest attainable aim,

But do not put up resistance in vain.

So far as possible, I myself have followed this philosophy, and it has made my life a happy one. Frankly, in looking back, I realize that I have not always succeeded to perfection, but this has been due to my own shortcomings, not those of the philosophy. As I have often said, 'The builder of the best racing car is not necessarily its best driver.'

Stress-related conditions

Key features and remedies

Key features	Remedy
Facial twitches and tics, especially if developed after a fright, shock or trauma, or if based on fear of events.	ACONITE
Feelings of extreme anxiety leading up to an event where the individual will be giving a presentation or will be the centre of attention.	ARGENT. NIT.
Feelings of extreme restlessness, often exhibited by the inability to remain still and to constantly tidy and fuss.	ARSEN. ALB.
Feeling that the body is in spasm. Mouth may twitch or there may be a coppery taste in the mouth.	CUPRUM MET.
Exhibits body tremors and shaking when frightened.	GELSEMIUM
Becomes hypersensitive to criticism, especially if involved in creative activities.	PHOSPHORUS
Suppression of emotions and anger. Need to be in control. Fear of loss of self-control. Workaholic.	STAPHISAGRIA
May appear expressionless, but remains talkative. Craves company. Rapid mood changes. May become aggressive and jealous.	STRAMONIUM

Feeling down in the dumps

Sometimes being under stress because of work, home life, finances, and so on, can make a client feel 'down in the dumps', an expression generally relating to feelings of lethargy and sadness, but stopping short of depression. In these cases a remedy may be selected that will influence a more positive state of mind. These remedies are very useful for individuals who may not wish to become self-analytical and do not wish, at the first stages of prescribing, to fully examine the nature of their stress.

Key features and remedies

Key features	Remedy
Loss of ambition, feelings of sadness and fear of failure in business.	ARGENT. NIT.
Body feels heavy and aching. Nothing will help to relieve the condition. Feels inadequate in their job.	ARNICA
Finds fault in everything, becomes irritable. Moans and groans a lot. Wants everything perfect and tidy.	ARSEN. ALB.
Feels sad and exhausted. In a rut. Does not want to move towards change. Can be moody and suspicious of help.	CALC. CARB.
General feelings of unhappiness and sadness. Hates work. May experience skin reactions (eczema, dryness, etc.).	GRAPHITES
Lives on their nerves. Feels weak and tired. Timid and self-conscious. Poor concentration and memory.	KALI PHOS.
Low self-confidence. Sadness on first waking. Puts a brave face on for work colleagues, but feels terrible once home. Mood swings.	LYCOPODIUM
Tired and burnt out. Avoids addressing problems. Avoids study or difficult work tasks. Needs reassurance. Oversensitivity to comments and remarks.	PHOSPHORUS
Irritable. Can become tearful and weeping. Moans about everything. Craves sympathy and attention. Changeable mood.	PULSATILLA
Easily offended. Miserable and irritable. Cries a lot. Lethargy. Fear of failure. Does not want to talk. Particularly when exhibited in women.	SEPIA

casestudy: Stress (female)

A young woman of 28 years came to see me, suffering from extreme anxiety and stress, which was manifesting itself in sleep problems, palpitations and tightness in the chest. After completing a detailed consultation, I discovered that this has started about a year ago while travelling to work on the tube train. She told me how she started to feel pain and tightness in her chest. The train was very overcrowded, but she did not normally suffer from claustrophobia. We talked about how she felt about herself at this point in her life and she told me that she had recently been through a relationship break-up and was not happy in her job. I could see that she had been living with a lot of simmering stress and tension and that it had reached boiling point on that particular journey to work. She went on to say that she was fearful of not finding a job that made her happy and of not meeting the right person to have a relationship with. When I questioned her further about how her last relationship had ended, she said it was due to her lack of trust, causing her to be suspicious and jealous of her boyfriend, even though he had never given her any reason to be. It came to light that she could be jealous in nature, especially of friends who had good jobs and relationships and were happy.

I could already begin to see a remedy picture emerging, based on the symptoms and the constitutional focus.

During our consultation she was very talkative, and when I asked her about her confidence in a social setting she said that she loved to talk and meet up with people. I asked her if she did most of the talking when meeting up with friends and she replied that she did. Before these conditions had manifested her health had not been good and she had been to her doctor to seek advice. The doctor referred her for a number of tests, such as ECG (electrocardiograph) for heart rate, and none of the results had indicated any heart problems. She was prone to the occasional cough or cold that always started with a sore throat. She mentioned that the sore throat was always the worst symptom and that it was her only 'vulnerable' area. She reported suffering from several sore throats each year and that they all cleared up naturally after no more than a few days. When I asked about clothing around her neck she said that she could not bear anything that restricted her neck, such as polo-neck sweaters, scarves, and so on. I found this an interesting point for an individual who enjoyed talking a lot (her job had little of this as she worked with computers). I could see she had become frustrated in her life and felt trapped and constricted. She was working and living her life, but felt panicked and fearful on the inside.

The symptoms of palpitations and tightness in the chest were causing her to feel fearful, almost to the point where she felt she could die. She felt the symptoms more on the left side, and when trying to sleep at night. Her whole body seemed to become tenser even when she was only describing the symptoms. She was also frustrated that the symptoms were unpredictable and that she could have 'good weeks and bad weeks'. This made her angry with herself. The palpitations would start to improve if she stopped moving, but any form of motion (e.g. on the tube train) would make the palpitations worse. The symptoms would also be worse for heat. Physically she was of slim to thin build.

To give some immediate relief, to help her with the anxiety about her future and to help with her restlessness, fear and panic, as well as to improve her sleep and alleviate palpitations, I prescribed Aconite. This remedy is not always good for chronic conditions as it is usually used when there is a sudden onset. She had been having the symptoms on and off for about a year, but when they did manifest it was with a sudden onset, so I judged the remedy would be of great therapeutic effect in this situation. Aconite is also a good remedy when the guiding symptom is fear, to the point where there is fear of death (even though the reality of death is unlikely), and tension and anxiety are prevalent, with much restlessness. I suggested one tablet in the 30c potency, three times a day, the first tablet to be taken in the morning before her journey to work, the second before her journey home and the third 20 minutes before bedtime. This was to be followed for three days, and if there was an improvement it could be reduced to two tablets a day, one before her journey and one at night before bed. This routine could then be continued for five days until her follow-up appointment. Aconite has the ability to 'bring down' a person from a heightened state, giving a calming effect and helping to remove fearfulness and thus prevent palpitations. The effect of this remedy can be very fast, and I am always amazed at how quickly it can bring about a positive result, in some cases even after just one dose.

On her second appointment (one week later) she reported that her sleep was improving and that she also felt better in herself for unloading her feelings during the last session. She said she was still having some palpitations, but that it felt more like a tightness in her chest and her reaction to it was not the usual one of panic and fear, and that it passed more quickly than usual. She also commented that after several days of taking the remedy she felt a little more 'peaceful' and less 'trapped'. She said if the improvements were to continue she would be happy to take the Aconite for the rest of her life! I told her that this was not the idea, and that once total improvement had been achieved it was a sign to stop taking the remedy, as it would have done its job. I felt we had reached a stage where Aconite had opened the door for the most needed remedy – Lachesis. This would work well as a constitutional remedy as it matched with likes, dislikes, personality and physical build. I suggested following the Aconite with Lachesis in a 30c potency, one tablet twice a day, once before travel and once before bedtime, for five to seven days. We would then meet again for a follow-up appointment.

At the follow-up appointment she reported that she could not believe how well the Lachesis had worked. The constriction and tightness she had experienced in her chest had felt 'freed', almost like a tight elastic band had released. She also said she was sleeping much better. One interesting point she made was that she felt angry with herself for not moving on in her life (e.g. finding a new job); this is a classic sign that Lachesis had worked as it is a known remedy for releasing feelings in the individual. I decided to give her a higher dose of Lachesis, three tablets of 200c. The tablets were to be taken at night, in the morning and then again at night. I prescribed this because a higher dose, for a short period, can help reach a further curative effect. I advised she take this after several days' break from the current 30c prescription, and then see me again in one month.

When I saw her next she was doing really well. She had the occasional feeling of tension, but no palpitations or tightness in the chest. I suggested we repeat the Lachesis, with a higher dose of 1m, in the same doses as before, as this would work well on a mental, emotional and constitutional level. It would help with her feelings of jealousy and suspicion, as often these symptoms are caused from the break-up of relationships. She agreed to take this increased dose. I saw her again one month later for a final session. She was feeling happy and well and also reported that she had been to several interviews for new jobs, and was more confident and relaxed 'in her own body'. I suggested that if she had a reoccurrence of the palpitations, or of feeling anxious and fearful, that she take the Aconite 30c immediately, and to always have this with her to help relieve any symptoms and help her to calm down. I also suggested that if the tightness in the chest was to reoccur she should take Lachesis 30c straight away. We spoke on the telephone a month later and I am pleased to report that she had only used the Aconite twice during this period, to help with her sleep. I feel the remedy selection had truly got to the heart and soul of this patient, and that this, in turn, had relieved her physical symptoms.

casestudy: Stress (male)

This man (28 years) had just moved house and was renovating a beautiful Victorian cottage. The builders had started work on this major renovation project several months before, with work including re-plastering, rewiring, heating, new bathrooms, and so on. It was no surprise that this man reported feeling an incredible amount of stress, particularly as he was living amid the renovations! He admitted to being very emotionally involved in the whole project due to his creative and passionate nature. He felt he was now paying the price, by experiencing tightness in the chest and palpitations, which at times made him think that he might be on the brink of a heart attack and death.

As well as the renovation project, he also worked as a therapist at a local complementary health clinic, practising aromatherapy, massage and reflexology. He was also a tutor of these therapies. He reported waking up one morning and thinking, *Physician, heal thyself*, at which point he made an appointment to see Nigel, the homeopath at the clinic where he worked. After going through a long consultation, covering what felt like every aspect of his life, he was initially prescribed Aconite in 30c potency. The results were almost magical, as he could not believe how much better he felt after taking the first few doses, with improved sleep and less tightness in the chest. The palpitations disappeared and he felt he had been rescued.

This man was Andrew James! I knew from that moment that I had to understand more about homeopathy, so I continued with several more treatments that treated me on a constitutional level. I then decided to study homeopathy. Nigel was such an inspiration. During and after my training I also had the privilege to work with Dr Christine Page, who went on to become a wonderful friend and mentor and provided me with even more reasons to become a homeopath.

FAQs: Stress

There seem to be a lot of remedies for stress and anxiousness. Which would be right for me?

By looking at the list of remedies in Chapter 3, select the remedies that are the closest match for your key features, then see if these fit your type in the list of constitutional types in Chapter 2 in order to narrow the choice further, depending on your modalities (personality, likes, dislikes, etc.). For example, tightness in the chest may have two different remedies, depending on the other factors:

- Tightness in the chest, with stress and palpitations, suppressed anger and feelings of constriction, made worse by touch and when sleeping. This might also be accompanied by jealousy and not being able to wear tight clothing around the neck. By taking into account all these factors, the best remedy would be Lachesis.

- Tightness in the chest, with stress and palpitations, accompanied by great fear of death. Symptoms arrive quickly and give feelings of loss of control and fear. Sleep is difficult. May feel better when outdoors. By taking into account all these factors, the best remedy would be Aconite.

8

pregnancy and homeopathy

Full-term pregnancy is usually 40 weeks from conception to birth. Signs that indicate a possible pregnancy are: missing a period, mild feelings of sickness and nausea, swollen and tender breasts, fatigue, passing urine more frequently, cravings for certain foods or a loss of appetite. A home pregnancy kit can confirm a pregnancy initially, but it is best to consult a doctor. Once confirmed by a doctor, it is necessary to register for antenatal care, check-ups, scans, and so on.

Homeopathy can be used pre-conception, as a constitutional treatment for the mother and father, through to birth (Arnica for pain relief, Aconite for fear, etc.) and beyond. Some common conditions relating to pregnancy are explored below.

Backache

Description of condition

An aching sensation, often localized in the lower back, but can be reported elsewhere along the spine. Lower back ache is common in pregnancy due to extra weight gain and the stretching of ligaments in the pelvic region.

Key features and remedies

Key features	Remedy
From injury (e.g. lifting and straining), with a bruised feeling.	ARNICA
Tense, vulnerable feeling in the lower back. Feels sensitive and tearful.	PULSATILLA
Stiffness, which improves with movement.	RHUS TOX.

Other information

Topical use of oil balm to the affected area. Arnica and Rhus Tox. balms are the most effective.

Constipation

Description of condition

A condition in which bowel movements happen less frequently than is normal for the particular individual, or the stool is small, hard and difficult or painful to pass.

Key features and remedies

Key features	Remedy
Hard and dry stools, mainly in the morning.	BRYONIA
With much wind. Small hard stools.	LYCOPODIUM
Uncomfortable, full feeling. Straining to pass stools.	NUX VOMICA
Hard, dry and large stools. Much pain in the rectum. May feel like a shooting pain.	SEPIA
With piles and hard, dry stools. Never feels bowels are completely emptied.	SULPHUR

Cystitis

Description of condition

A bladder infection, marked by pain, as well as frequent, painful urination. In the case of pregnancy, it may be due to extreme pressure to the bladder and weak pelvic muscles.

Key features and remedies

Key features	Remedy
At the first stages. Anxious and restless.	ACONITE
Sore, stinging and burning pain. Pain before, during and after passing urine.	CANTHARIS
When lying down in bed. Slight leakage.	PULSATILLA
Discomfort after passing urine. Burning and stinging sensation. Need to pass urine throughout the night.	SULPHUR

Emotional problems

Description of condition

Emotional problems can cover a wide variety of psychological problems, from feeling low to depression, anxiety and insomnia.

Key features and remedies

Key features	Remedy
Fear, great anxiety. Tightness in the chest. Palpitations. Worries all the time. Whole body feels tense.	ACONITE
Bad-tempered. Critical of loved ones. Very irritable.	NUX VOMICA
Very fearful and sensitive. Imagination runs wild.	PHOSPHORUS
Tearful, weeps easily. Very sensitive to criticism. Feeling sorry for yourself.	PULSATILLA

Haemorrhoids/piles

Description of condition

Enlarged veins in the anus or rectum, generally caused by constipation or straining to have a bowel movement. Very common in pregnancy or after childbirth.

Key features and remedies

Key features	Remedy
Burning pain after passing a stool. Strained external veins.	CARBO VEG.
Sharp, cutting pain.	CHAMOMILLA
Aching, burning with sore and heavy sensations.	HAMAMELIS (can be used as a topical cream to ease localized discomfort)
With constipation.	NUX VOMICA
Sore and sensitive.	PULSATILLA

High blood pressure

Description of condition

Persistent elevation of blood pressure above the normal range. Often due to anxiety. Seek help from GP immediately.

Key features and remedies

Key features	Remedy
With anxiousness and fear. Palpitations.	ACONITE
Feeling weak and emotional. Tearful and weeping.	PULSATILLA

In labour

Description of condition

The beginning of labour feels different for every woman. Labour is indicated by frequent and regular contractions. The length of labour varies for all women. The average labour lasts 12–14 hours for a first baby. Labour is often faster for second and subsequent children.

Key features and remedies

Key features	Remedy
Feels battered and bruised. Aches all over.	ARNICA
Full of anguish and fear. Very hot and throbbing.	BELLADONNA
Normal labour, painful contractions. Restless.	COFFEA
Feels very impatient. Feels like wanting to urinate constantly or pass a stool.	NUX VOMICA
Very restless and tearful. Sensitive and needs a lot of reassurance. Slowness to labour. Feels exhausted.	PULSATILLA

Morning sickness

Description of condition

Nausea and vomiting experienced early in a pregnancy, affecting about half of all pregnant women. Most common in the second and third months, and may not be in the morning only.

Key features and remedies

Key features	Remedy
Nausea and diarrhoea. Feeling fatigued and restless.	ARSEN. ALB.
Sickness, with craving for salty foods and a great thirst.	NAT. MUR.
Feelings of sickness. Wanting to vomit in the morning.	NUX VOMICA
Feelings of sickness later in the day. Feeling better by the evening. Feels vulnerable and tearful.	PULSATILLA
Vomiting, with feelings of sadness. Weeping and tearful.	SEPIA

Postnatal depression

Description of condition

After giving birth, some women experience an episode of 'baby blues' – feelings of depression, anger, anxiety and guilt, lasting for several days. About 10 per cent of new mothers develop the more severe postnatal depression, a form of major depression which requires medical treatment.

Key features and remedies

Key features	Remedy
Wants to be left alone. Becomes withdrawn. Feelings of guilt. Cannot be consoled.	NAT. MUR.
Very tearful. Weeps easily. Sensitive and sad.	PULSATILLA
Lack of interest in surroundings. Tired and irritable. Happy throughout pregnancy, but becomes low afterwards.	SEPIA

Sleep problems

Description of condition

Difficulty in getting to sleep through anxiousness. Constant waking due to the need to urinate. Lower back discomfort. Difficulty in finding a comfortable position to sleep in.

Key features and remedies

Key features	Remedy
Feeling anxious and afraid. Cannot switch off.	ACONITE
Mind is overstimulated and overexcited – 'can't wait'.	COFFEA
Fear of previous miscarriage or complications. Fear of loss of baby.	IGNATIA

Sore breasts

Description of condition

One of the early signs of pregnancy is extremely sensitive, sore breasts, due to hormonal changes in the body. Some women's breasts become so sensitive, in fact, that the sensation of a nightgown against them is unbearable. It can also occur during the last stages of pregnancy, with milk formation.

Key features and remedies

Key features	Remedy
Feeling bruised and aching.	ARNICA
Hard, swollen and tight, with red streaking of the skin.	BELLADONNA
Breasts feel hard and tight.	BRYONIA

Stress incontinence

Description of condition

Stress incontinence is a condition in which urine leaks when a person coughs, sneezes, laughs, exercises, lifts heavy objects or does anything that puts pressure on the bladder, often due to weak muscles in the pelvic floor and the pressure of pregnancy.

Key features and remedies

Key features	Remedy
Triggered by walking and movement. Sometimes cannot feel leakage.	CAUSTICUM
Slight leakage. Need to urinate urgently. No symptoms of cystitis. Experiences a dragging, 'bearing down' sensation.	SEPIA

Varicose veins

Description of condition

Enlarged, twisted, painful, superficial veins, resulting from poorly functioning valves. Seen most often in the legs (also called varicosities), although they can be found in other parts of the body. Usually they appear as lumpy, winding vessels just below the surface of the skin. Extreme weight may put a strain on the pelvic veins. Existing varicose veins may become more agitated and distended.

Key features and remedies

Key features	Remedy
Skin feels tight and looks shiny. A 'marble' look to the skin. Painful.	CARBO VEG.
Burning and stinging sensations. Heavy, aching feeling.	HAMAMELIS
With backache and heaviness in the legs. Aching veins. Better for elevation and rest.	PULSATILLA

FAQs: Pregnancy and babies

Is it safe to take homeopathic remedies while pregnant?

Yes, but it is advisable to consult your doctor or pharmacist before purchasing a remedy, and always consult your doctor if you are suffering from any medical condition during pregnancy. When using topical applications, always read the label carefully and follow the instructions for use in pregnancy. If unsure, check with the manufacturer of the product. Often the homeopathic supplier will have a pharmacist on hand who can give advice and guidance.

Is it okay to give the homeopathic remedies to young children and babies?

Yes. It is easier to give the remedies in soft tablets or powder form, as these dissolve easier on contact with saliva, and this makes it difficult to spit them out. Soft tablets can also be crushed into a powder by placing the tablets on a clean piece of paper and crushing them with a spoon; then you can shape the paper into a funnel and tap the powder into the mouth. It is only necessary to wait 20 minutes after giving the remedy before eating or drinking. Ainsworths (homeopathic pharmacy) supply soft tablets and powders to order. If you are wishing to treat babies or children, it is advisable to purchase a book aimed at treating their common conditions (there are many available).

travel and first aid kit

When compiling a homeopathic travel kit, the choice of remedies will be dependent on the type of travel involved and the reasons for it (e.g. travelling to a funeral by aeroplane will require a different approach to travelling on holiday in a car). Each circumstance will result in different emotional and physical reactions.

Aircraft travel for holidays is one of the most common forms of travel. To prescribe for this the homeopath needs to establish if there is a fear of flying, resulting in outward displays of nervousness and worry that may build up gradually, long before the date of travel, or if there are more obvious displays of acute fear and extreme anxiety, such as disrupted sleep patterns, bowel disturbance IBS (irritable bowel syndrome), severe headaches, neck pain, skin breakouts such as eczema, dermatitis or acne, sweating and increased blood pressure. All these symptoms need to be treated with reference to the behaviour pattern of the individual. For example, if the individual begins to become nervous a week before the flight, this is the time to start the remedies. (A guide to selecting the appropriate remedies appears below.) During the flight itself legs can ache and become swollen, sleep may be disrupted and cramp and constipation may be evident. A feeling of claustrophobia can also be common. Once again, remedies should be selected which reflect these symptoms.

Other common forms of physical and emotional imbalance associated with many forms of travel, such as trains, boats and cars, are 'sea sickness', dizziness, backache, noise

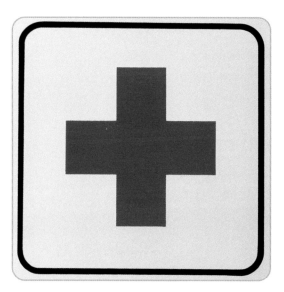

sensitivity, anxiety, swollen ankles and irritability.

Once at a destination, symptoms of jet lag, disorientation, tiredness, dehydration, tired and aching limbs, blocked sinuses, headaches and earache can all be felt long after the journey has come to an end. During the stay it would be advisable to have remedies to help with specific common problems, such as sunburn, insect bites and stings, upset stomach, constipation or diarrhoea, insomnia,

cuts and grazes. In a cold climate, remedies for chilblains, frostbite and blisters are also useful. If a holiday involves vigorous exercise, such as hiking or skiing, remedies for muscular aches and pains would also be vital.

In prescribing a remedy it is best to recall how your body has reacted to past travel experiences and situations in order to help identify the areas that will need treating. This includes remedies for overindulgence, such as hangovers and indigestion!

Backache

Key features and remedies

Key features	Remedy
Heavy and aching, with a bruised feeling.	ARNICA
Great stiffness. Feels need to move and adjust constantly. Suffers from cramp.	RHUS TOX.

Bites and stings

Key features and remedies

Key features	Remedy
Burning and stinging pain.	CANTHARIS
Itching pain. Scratching makes it worse. Visible puncture wound.	LEDUM

Other information

Topical applications of Calendula and Hypericum (mix) in lotion or spray for bites and stings can help relieve some of the symptoms.

Blisters

Key features and remedies

Key features	Remedy
Burning, itching and sore.	CANTHARIS
Bleeding and weeping if burnt.	HYPERICUM
Very itchy blisters, red and swollen skin around the blister.	RHUS TOX.

Circulation (aching legs and feet, swollen ankles, etc.)

Key features and remedies

Key features	Remedy
Cramp, particularly in the toes. Constricting, cramp-like symptoms in the legs.	CUPRUM MET.
Legs feel heavy, sore, aching and burning. Irritated varicose veins. Feelings of bruising.	HAMAMELIS
Heavy, aching limbs. Shoes or trainers feel tight to wear.	LACHESIS
Feels legs need to be raised. Legs feel worse if lowered. Excellent remedy if pregnant.	PULSATILLA
Restless legs, cramp and with varicose veins present. May feel chilly.	ZINC. MET.

Other information

Topical creams, gel and sprays are useful before and during travel. Flight socks will help during long periods of sedentary travel. Avoid alcohol and heavy meals while travelling, particularly on an aircraft.

Fear experienced before or during travel

Key features and remedies

Key features	Remedy
A first-choice remedy for fear associated with travel of any kind. It may be a sudden onset of shock, with palpitations, which may then subside into restlessness and anxiety. Panic attacks and irrational fear are also a clear indicator. Fears about safety and health, often accompanied by nightmares, also respond well to this remedy.	ACONITE
For general anxiousness and for becoming fussy and restless during a journey.	ARSEN. ALB.
For irritability and sleeplessness before or during a journey. The traveller may also become more irritable for lack of sleep, which creates a vicious circle.	BRYONIA
For the traveller who is very self-conscious and feels everyone is looking at them. This makes them feel more sensitive and anxious, often accompanied by wringing and fidgeting of the hands.	CALC. CARB.
For exhaustion resulting from panic attacks and worry. It can be manifested not only as exhaustion, but also as trembling, flu-like symptoms.	GELSEMIUM
This remedy is known as the great nerve soother. It is useful for people with a nervous disposition. It also works well for those whose fear and panic is suppressed initially, but works up over a period of days until it peaks in a near-hysterical state. In this case, the remedy is best started several days before any travel, particularly if early symptoms begin – such as anxiousness, loose bowels and increased sweating.	KALI PHOS.
Ideal for fear of travelling alone, and of restlessness and agitation when travelling. It also helps with fear of storms and increased sensitivity to events surrounding the individual. Tight chests and hoarse or dry throats also respond well to this remedy.	PHOSPHORUS

Heat stroke

Key features and remedies

Key features	Remedy
Sun-induced, throbbing pain, with pounding headache. Flushed skin. Head hurts if moved.	BELLADONNA
Thirsty and chilly. Severe headache. Needs to keep head still. Nausea.	BRYONIA

Sunburn

Key features and remedies

Key features	Remedy
If mild, then use this for first two or three doses.	ARNICA
Red and throbbing, with much heat.	BELLADONNA
Stinging and burning skin. Remedy of choice if also suffering from insect bites or stings.	CANTHARIS

Other information

Topical applications of Arnica cream can also ease the condition. Good quality aloe vera gel is also useful.

Travel sickness

Key features and remedies

Key features	Remedy
Worse for seeing or smelling food. Vomiting. Sickness during pregnancy.	ARSEN. ALB.
Constantly feeling sick. General travel sickness. Still feels sick, even after vomiting.	IPECAC.
Sickness, with headaches and feeling queasy.	NUX VOMICA
During pregnancy.	PULSATILLA

Other information

Start to take the remedy one hour before travel if you know that you are likely to experience the symptoms.

Homeopathic first aid kit

A homeopathic first aid kit is a very useful item to have around the house, in the car or

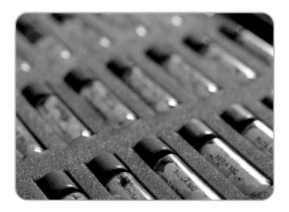

on holiday. Several homeopathic pharmacies/suppliers can provide a ready-made first aid kit, often consisting of about 18 remedies in small bottles or vials. It may not be necessary for your kit to contain this many remedies, of course; take a look at the remedies listed in Chapter 3 and decide which ones would be of most use to you and your family. You may have used some of the remedies already and/or worked out your constitutional remedy, and therefore know which ones work well for you. To help you decide which to include there are several highlighted as possible first aid kit remedies under the remedy listings in the same chapter.

You may wish to purchase a small remedy box in which to store your customized first aid kit. Ten remedies would normally be sufficient, consisting of some of the following suggestions. Also remember to include your constitutional remedy and any remedy relating to an existing condition.

First aid remedies

Key feature	Remedy
For panic. Fear. Pain. First signs of a cold or sore throat and fever. Inability to relax. Anxiety. To help with inducing sleep after a long journey. Any condition with a sudden onset.	ACONITE
For bites and stings. Fluid retention and swelling. Swelling of legs and feet with travel.	APIS MEL.
Shock. Injury. Bruising. Neck, back, shoulder and joint pain. Sprains and strains. Headaches.	ARNICA (topical application of Arnica cream or ointment for bruising, sprains and strains; sunburn – not to be applied if skin is broken)
Chronic cystitis. Burning, stinging pain. Insect bites and stings. Sunburn.	CANTHARIS
Sore throats. Coughs and colds. Influenza with shivering.	GELSEMIUM

Allergies. Reactions or breakouts of the skin due to change of climate or change of washing powder, and so on. Reactions to swimming pool chemicals. Eczema. Dermatitis.	GRAPHITES (topical application of cream to calm, soothe and treat eczema, dermatitis or itchy, irritated skin)
Puncture wounds. Splinters. Bites and stings.	LEDUM
Food poisoning. Travel sickness. Upset stomach. Jet lag. Hangover. Overindulgence of rich foods.	NUX VOMICA
Muscular aches and pains. Stiffness and overexertion. Back and joint pain. Muscular aches and pains. Useful after skiing/trekking or activity holidays.	RHUS TOX. (topical application of Rhus Tox. for muscular aches and pains; backaches; after sport, and so on)

Other information

Hypericum/Calendula pre-mixed cream, ointment or tincture: for cleaning of cuts and wounds; ointment or cream for application on wounds, cuts and grazes or insect bites and stings.

Bach flower rescue remedy

Although the Bach flower remedies are not homeopathic remedies, they are based on Dr Bach's system of healing. Dr Bach was a Harley Street doctor in the 1930s who practised homeopathy. He devised a system of seven emotional groups, consisting of fear, loneliness, uncertainty, overcare for others, depression/despair, oversensitivity and insufficient interest in present circumstances. He developed natural remedies, diluted in brandy, to treat these groupings.

For the purposes of the first aid kit, the Bach flower rescue remedy is a useful addition. The rescue remedy is a combination of the five remedies: rock rose for terror, clematis for lack of interest, cherry plum for fear, impatiens for impatience and star of Bethlehem for shock. The rescue remedy can be used by diluting four drops in a small glass of water or it can be applied directly to the tongue. It is excellent in a first aid situation for shock, extreme anxiety and fear. It can be used alongside homeopathic remedies in a first aid situation.

FAQs: First aid

Which is best when buying remedies – pills, tablets, soft tablets or powders? Are some easier to take or quicker to work?

Most remedies available are in tablet form, especially those found in health food stores and chemists. 'Pilules' are sometimes available, which are smaller, round, hard pills. Both types are suitable for most remedies and conditions in adults. For children I would recommend soft tablets, as these dissolve instantly on the tongue and the waiting time before consuming food or drink afterwards is reduced to approximately 15–20 minutes. Soft tablets are also a good choice for a first aid kit, due to their quick dissolving nature and the fact that it may be necessary to repeat the remedy at shorter intervals. Soft tablets are also useful where a condition means that sucking the harder tablets causes pain or discomfort, such as mouth ulcers and sore throats. If it is not possible to obtain soft tablets, hard tablets can be crushed into a powder by placing the tablets in paper and crushing with the back of a spoon. The crushed tablets must be funnelled into the mouth from the paper.

I am travelling and want to put a small kit together – what remedies would you recommend?

Obtain a small wallet in which to carry the remedies (these are available from most homeopathic suppliers). I would include Arnica, Aconite, Nux Vomica, Cantharis and Hypericum. Aconite is excellent for the sudden onset of most conditions and is also good for shock and sleep problems. Arnica is excellent for bruises and aches and pains, and aids healing. Cantharis is good for stings, bites and sunburn. Hypericum is good for infections of wounds and cuts and has an anti-inflammatory effect. Nux Vomica will help with feelings of sickness, food poisoning, hangovers and upset stomachs. I would obtain Arnica and Aconite in soft tablets if you have children. I would also try to include a tincture of Calendula and Hypericum, which can be useful for bathing wounds or for inflamed skin, sore feet and blisters.

Can I buy ready-made homeopathic first aid kits?

Yes. Many homeopathic suppliers offer kits that consist of anything from 10 to 42 remedies, supplied in a carry case or wallet. (Ainsworths homeopathic pharmacy have an excellent range.)

topical applications and combination remedies

Topical applications

When using topical applications always read the label carefully and follow the instructions, especially if using when pregnant. If you are unsure, check with the manufacturer of the product and consult your doctor. Often the homeopathic supplier will also have a pharmacist on hand who can give advice and guidance.

Some homeopathic remedies can also be used in mediums that are applied directly to the skin (known as topical applications), for example creams, lotions, ointments, tinctures, sprays and massage balms. These topical applications are an ideal way to back up the oral remedies, on their own or as a first aid treatment. The following are the most commonly available and can be purchased ready-mixed.

Arnica

- Bruising, muscular aches and pains.
- Sprains and strains.
- After sport or exercise.
- Joint pain.
- Aching, stiff back.
- Tired, aching feet.
- First signs of RSI (repetitive strain injury).
- Frozen shoulder.
- Neck pain and stiffness.
- Sunburn (do not apply to broken skin).

Calendula

- Sensitive, dry, irritated and inflamed skin.
- Acne.
- Contact dermatitis.

- Eczema.
- Rashes.
- Cradle cap.
- Dandruff and scalp problems.
- Dry, cracked and sore skin, including ears and lips.
- Cold sores.
- Fungal infections.
- To clean cuts and wounds.
- As a facial moisturizer or aftershave balm.
- Razor burn.
- Sunburn.
- On babies' skin, for minor irritations such as nappy rash and grazes.
- Boils and abscesses.

Euphrasia

- Conjunctivitis, sensitivity to bright light.
- Dry eyes, eye injuries and inflammation.
- Hay fever that affects the eyes.
- Watery, stinging discharge from the eyes.

Hypericum

- Cuts, sores, wounds, scrapes and grazes.
- Cold sores.
- Itchy, irritated and inflamed skin, including acne.
- Splinters.
- Nail irritations (nail-bed cuts or bitten, sore nails).
- Cracked, sore lips.
- Blisters.

- Sore, bleeding haemorrhoids (external).
- Dandruff and scalp problems.
- Boils and abscesses.
- Cystitis.

Graphites

- Eczema.
- Contact dermatitis.
- Psoriasis.
- Varicose eczema, or to help prevent this condition where skin is dry, thin and translucent.
- Extremely dry, itchy, sore skin.
- Sore skin in and around the nose, accompanied by a cold.
- Cold sores.
- Facial moisturizer to help clear eczema, dermatitis or allergic reaction to cosmetics.

Hamamelis

- Sore, burning, itchy skin.
- Varicose veins.
- Phlebitis.
- Haemorrhoids.
- Heavy, aching legs and feet, in particular after long periods of standing (always apply lightly around varicose sites; do not use on broken skin).

Rhus Tox.

- Muscular aches and pains, in particular from overexertion (gardening, housework, sport, etc.).

- RSI (repetitive strain injury).
- Joint pain (tennis elbow and knee injuries).
- Arthritis and rheumatism.
- Sciatica.
- Useful to use after Arnica, once the bruising has diminished.
- Do not apply to broken skin.

Ruta Grav.

- Stiffness and pain in tendons, ligaments, joints and muscles, where there is a deep aching.
- RSI (repetitive strain injury).
- Sciatica.
- Rib and chest pain during and after coughs to help heal muscle strain.
- Good for ankle and wrist pain where there has been overuse through sport.
- Do not apply to broken skin.

Thuja

- Warts.
- Verrucas.
- Brittle, weak nails.

When deciding to use cream, ointment, tincture, massage balm or spray, you should consider the following.

Creams

Creams will sink into the skin well and will not leave a greasy, sticky after-feeling. They are ideal for the face, hands and feet and when clothing has to be worn directly after application.

Ointments

Ointments are more greasy and lubricating, which makes then ideal for light, gentle massage into the affected muscles and joints. They are useful if resting directly afterwards or if covering with a dressing. Ointments will cover a larger area than creams due to the gliding effect of the mixture.

Tinctures

Tinctures are liquids and so are useful for cleaning cuts, grazes, scrapes and wounds. They are also useful as part of a cool or warm compress. Always add the tincture to boiled water that has been cooled or left until warm. Mix 20 drops of tincture to approximately 0.5 pint of water. If using two tinctures (e.g. Hypericum and Calendula), use 10 drops of each. Tinctures are also useful for foot and hand baths, and can also be used in a normal bath by adding 30 drops to the bath water once run. With Euphrasia tincture, use as an eye bath only – 20 drops to 0.5 pint of warm water, up to four times a day – or soak on tissue pads to lie over the eyes.

Massage balms

Usually the homeopathic remedy is carried in a vegetable oil base. Massage balms are useful for muscular aches and pains, back stiffness and pain and where gentle massage and rubbing helps improve the condition. They are excellent for sportspeople and gardeners, and can be used as a preventative measure if an individual is prone to aches and pains. The most commonly available ready-made massage balms are Arnica, Calendula and Rhus Tox. Calendula massage balm is of particular benefit when massaging babies and young children, or adults with sensitive skin with a tendency to become inflamed or irritated.

Sprays

Sprays are usually available ready-mixed for treating insect bites and stings (Pyrethrum spray). A do-it-yourself spray can be made by following the same mixing instructions as detailed under Tinctures (above), with Calendula and Arnica for sunburn or Hamamelis for hot, swollen varicose veins (the spray is best kept cool in the fridge prior to application). A nasal spray, Rhinodoron, is also available from Weleda (supplier of homeopathic medicines and natural body-care products); it is aloe vera-based and clears, moisturizes and reduces inflammation in the nasal passages. It is useful for sinus problems, coughs, colds, hay fever and allergic reactions.

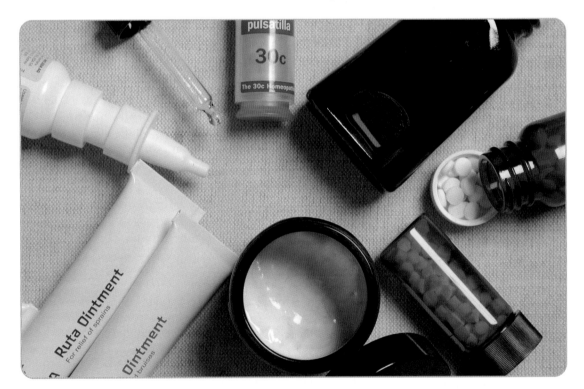

Combination remedies
(recommended by the author)

Aurum Met./lavender/rose ointment (supplied on request by Weleda)

This is useful for panic attacks, anxiety, depression, anorexia, sleep disturbance, nightmares, insomnia and stress. Apply the ointment to the heart area with gentle, circular, clockwise movements using your fingertips, for several minutes. Repeat night and morning. This helps balance and soothe the mind and body, and lift feelings of self-worth and spirit. It is excellent for 'centring' an individual.

Skin tone lotion (supplied by Weleda)

This contains Arnica and other natural remedies. It refreshes and revitalizes circulation to tired, aching limbs. It has a gel-like consistency and can be used from the fridge in hot weather. It is non-stick, so clothes can be worn directly after an application. It is useful for treating varicose veins, fluid retention, restless legs and aching muscles. When applying any product over varicose veins, remember to do so lightly and gently – never rub over the veins; always smooth on in the direction of the venous flow (towards the heart).

Aesculus Hamamelis Paeonia cream (supplied by Ainsworths)

This is for varicose veins and circulatory conditions affecting the legs. It has a good moisturizing effect.

Frost cream (supplied by Weleda)

This contains Arnica, Petroleum and other natural remedies. It is used for the treatment of chilblains and Raynaud's disease. Massage into the fingers and toes, morning and night.

Dermatodoron ointment (supplied by Weleda)

This contains a mixture of natural-based remedies. It is used for the treatment of eczema. Apply to the affected area three to four times a day. It has a relieving effect on dry, stubborn eczema.

Oleum Rhinale drops (supplied by Weleda)

This is a homeopathic and essential oil-based liquid, to be used as nasal drops. Use two to four drops in each nostril. It is excellent for catarrh or sinus problems, hay fever and allergies.

Herbal aloe gold ear drops (supplied by Higher Nature, an online natural food store)

An aloe and herbal-based ear drop, it soothes and heals ear canals and gently creates the optimum pH balance that discourages bacteria and fungal infections. It is excellent for regular swimmers or those prone to recurring ear infections.

Medicinal gargle (supplied by Weleda)

This is a gargle containing homeopathic and other natural-based remedies. It relieves mouth ulcers, tender gums, gingivitis and sore throats. It can be used as a regular mouthwash for oral hygiene. Use 10–20 drops in 100 ml of cooled, warm water.

Avena sativa comp. drops (supplied by Weleda)

This is a homeopathic and natural-based remedy tincture, which calms and relaxes, and combats nervous irritability, restlessness, sleep problems, insomnia and teeth grinding. Use 10 drops in a small glass of water three times a day. At night use 20 drops 30 minutes before bedtime. It is an excellent remedy for promoting a regular sleep pattern and can be used regularly for up to one month.

Soap

For a natural soap, Calendula is an excellent choice (supplied by Ainsworths).

Toothpaste

Homeopathic-compatible toothpastes that do not contain mint or peppermint are available, such as Calendula toothpaste. Calendula toothpaste is always excellent for treatment of regular mouth ulcers or bleeding gums (available from Ainsworths or Weleda).

Cough mixture

Several homeopathic cough mixtures are available, such as Bryonia (available from Ainsworths or Weleda).

Tips

It may be useful to note that some pharmacies and suppliers of homeopathic medicines offer creams, ointments, tinctures, massage balms, and so on, ready-mixed to order. For example, Calendula and Hypericum may be supplied mixed together, avoiding the need to buy the two separately. It is also possible to have a topical application custom-made, using a remedy of your choice, on the advice of a homeopath or homeopathic pharmacy.

where to go from here

I f you have trouble obtaining your remedy from the pharmacist, chemist or health shop, try one of the suppliers listed below.

Most will supply ointments, creams, tinctures, and so on, as well as homeopathic tablets, boxes and carry cases.

Suppliers of homeopathic medicines

- Ainsworths Pharmacy
  36 New Cavendish Street
  London W1G 8UF
  www.ainsworths.com (accessed
  26 January 2006)

- Helios Homoeopathic Pharmacy
  97 Camden Road
  Tunbridge Wells
  Kent TN1 2QR
  www.helios.co.uk (accessed
  26 January 2006)

- Nelsons Homeopathic Pharmacy Mail
  Order
  73 Duke Street
  London W1K 5BY

  www.nelsonshomoeopathy.co.uk
  (accessed 26 January 2006)

- The Homeopathic Supply Company
  The Street
  Bodham
  Holt
  Norfolk NR25 6AD
  www.homeopathicsupply.com (accessed
  26 January 2006)

- Weleda (UK) Ltd
  Heanor Road
  Ilkeston
  Derbyshire DE7 8DR
  www.weleda.co.uk (accessed
  26 January 2006)

Suppliers of natural/herbal remedies and supplements

- Blackmores (UK)
  Naturopathic Health & Wellness Centres
  Blackmores Professional UK
  Holly House
  300–302 Chiswick High Road
  London W4 1NP

  www.blackmores.com (accessed 26 January 2006)

- Higher Nature
  Burwash Common
  East Sussex TN19 7LX
  www.highernature.co.uk (accessed 26 January 2006)

NHS homeopathic hospitals

- Bristol Homeopathic Hospital
  Cotham Hill
  Cotham
  Bristol BS6 6JU
  www.ubht.nhs.uk/homeopathy (accessed 26 January 2006)

- Glasgow Homeopathic Hospital
  1053 Great Western Road
  Glasgow G12 OXQ
  www.adhom.com (accessed 26 January 2006)

- The Royal London Homeopathic Hospital
  60 Great Ormond Street
  London WC1N 3HR
  www.rlhh.org.uk (accessed 26 January 2006)

- Tunbridge Wells Homeopathic Hospital
  Church Road
  Tunbridge Wells
  Kent TN1 1JU

Homeopathic organisations

For a register of medically qualified homeopaths:

- Alliance of Registered Homeopaths
  Millbrook
  Millbrook Hill
  Nutley
  East Sussex
  TN22 3PJ
  www.a-r-h.org

- British Homeopathic Association
  Hahnemann House
  29 Park Street West
  Luton LU1 3BE
  www.trusthomeopathy.org (accessed 26 January 2006)

For non-medically and medically qualified homeopaths:

- The Society of Homeopaths

  11 Brookfield

  Duncan Close

  Moulton Park

  Northampton NN3 6WL

  www.homeopathy-soh.org (accessed 26 January 2006)

- Homeopathic Medical Association – UK

  6 Livingstone Road

  Gravesend

  Kent DA12 5DZ

www.the-hma.org (accessed 26 January 2006)

- The British Institute of Homeopathy Ltd

  Endeavour House

  80 High Street

  Egham

  Surrey TW20 9HE

  www.britinsthom.com (accessed 26 January 2006)

Please note that some homeopaths prefer not to have their address or telephone number listed on registers. Always check the qualifications of your homeopath. **Personal recommendation is always the best way to find a good homeopath.**

Further reading

Homeopathy

Trevor Cook, 2000, third Edition British Institute of Homeopathy (ISBN 152228203)

Trevor Cook, 1981, *Samuel Hahnemann: Founder of Homoeopathic Medicine*, Thorsons (ISBN 0722506899).

Dr Andrew Lockie, 1998, *The Family Guide to Homeopathy*, Hamish Hamilton (ISBN 0241135729).

Dr Andrew Lockie and Dr Nicola Geddes, 2000, *The Complete Guide to Homeopathy: The Principles and Practice of Treatment*, DK Publishing (ISBN 0789459531).

George Vithoulkas, 2000, *The Science of Homoeopathy*, Grove Press/Atlantic Monthly Press (ISBN 0802151205).

Holistic

Louise L. Hay, 2003, *You Can Heal Your Life*, Full Circle Publishing Ltd (ISBN 8176210773).

Dr Christine R. Page, 2000, *Frontiers of Health: From Healing to Wholeness*, C.W. Daniel & Co. Ltd (ISBN 0852073402).

Other books by this author

Andrew James, 2002, *Hands On Reflexology*, Hodder Arnold (ISBN 0340803975).

Further training

For introductory workshops and courses up to foundation level, contact your local further or adult education college. Many private colleges also offer these courses. For a choice of colleges offering training to practitioner level, contact the various homeopathic bodies as listed under Homeopathic organizations, above. Some colleges, such as the British Institute of Homeopathy (www.britinsthom.com), offer specialist homeopathic training for dentists, pharmacists, vets, midwives, and so on.

Treatment or workshops and courses in complementary therapy with the author

The author can be contacted by email.

For clinic enquiries and bookings: **andrew@lmsltd.co.uk** (this is an appointment and consultation service in London only – the author regrets that individual health queries cannot be answered via this service).

For training and workshops: **info@ handsonreflexology.com** (website: www. handsonreflexology.com).

FAQs: Where to go from here

I want to help friends and family at home, but I do not want to study for a qualification – where do I go?

Once you have done some background reading and understand the basics, start with a one-day workshop. There are workshops available through local adult education centres. If you enjoy this, a short 6–10 week course may add to your learning experience and give you enough knowledge and confidence to help yourself and your loved ones. Always remember, if a condition does not improve or you are unsure about the cause of any symptoms, you should consult your doctor immediately.

I have really enjoyed learning about the remedies and their uses – where can I go from here?

You can study at a foundation level, available at many adult and further education colleges. This would enable you to treat family and friends and gain a stronger underpinning knowledge of the subject. Practitioner courses are also available, including open university-style correspondence courses. All practitioner courses require a clinical internship.

Glossary

Acute: A sudden onset of symptoms or disease

Chronic: A persistent and lasting condition

Condition: A state of health at a particular time

Constitution: Character of body, regarding health, strength and mental character

Diagnosis: The process of identifying a disease by its signs, symptoms and results of various diagnostic procedures. The conclusion reached through that process is also called a diagnosis.

Dilution: the act of making thinner or more liquid by adding to the mixture; the act of diminishing the strength.

Dosage: The amount of medication that one may take or use.

Emotions: A person's mental state of being, normally based in or tied to the person's internal (physical) and external (social) sensory feeling.

Essential oils: Aromatic oils extracted from the leaves, stems, flowers, and other parts of plants. Therapeutic use generally includes dilution of the highly concentrated oil.

Frequency: the number of occurrences within a given time period.

Inflammation: a response of body tissues to injury or irritation; characterized by pain and swelling and sometimes redness and heat.

Localised: confined or restricted to a particular location.

Modalities: Influences that worsen or improve the symptoms of the patient.

Tincture: Liquid remedies, ready for dilution.

Pillues: Small, round hard pills.

Potenisation: the strength of a homeopathic remedy

Proving: homeopathic proving is an experiment undertaken by a group of healthy individuals in order to test the medicinal effects of a particular substance.

Prescribe: A direction to be followed

Remedy: medicine, as in homeopathic remedy.

Succussion: The forceful shaking of liquid homeopathic remedies that allows the permeation of the original substance into the liquid medium.

Temperament: temperament is the general nature of an individual's personality, such as introversion or extraversion.

Topical: Any solution that is administered by applying it to the surface of the skin.

Vital force: The bodies own healing potential.

index